The Definitive Plant-Based Handbook

Delicious and Healthy Plant-Based Recipes to Boost Your Meals and Improve Your Diet

I0146052

Clay Palmer

Table of Contents

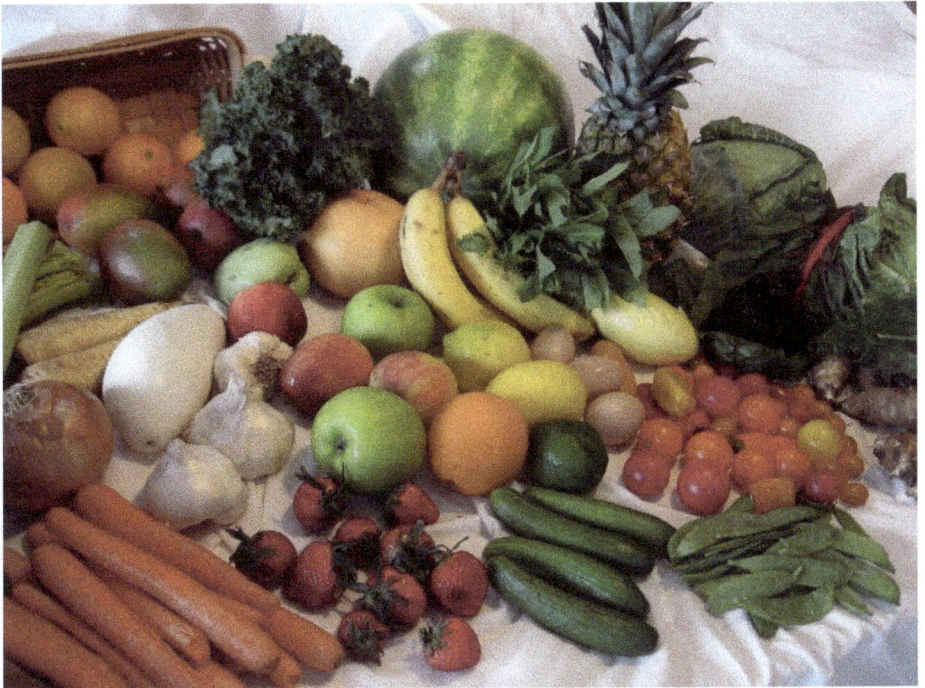

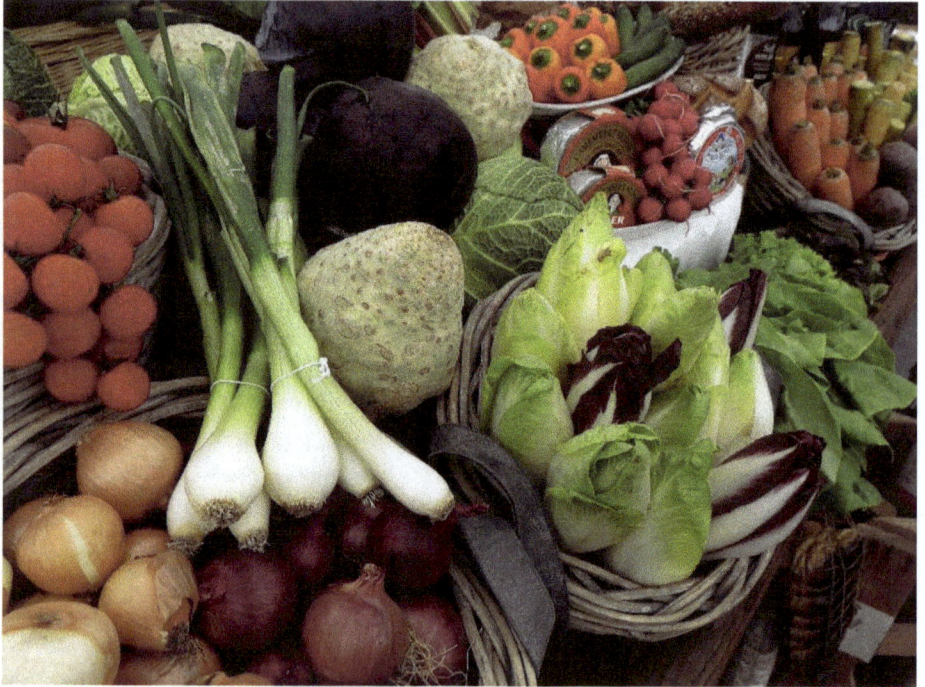

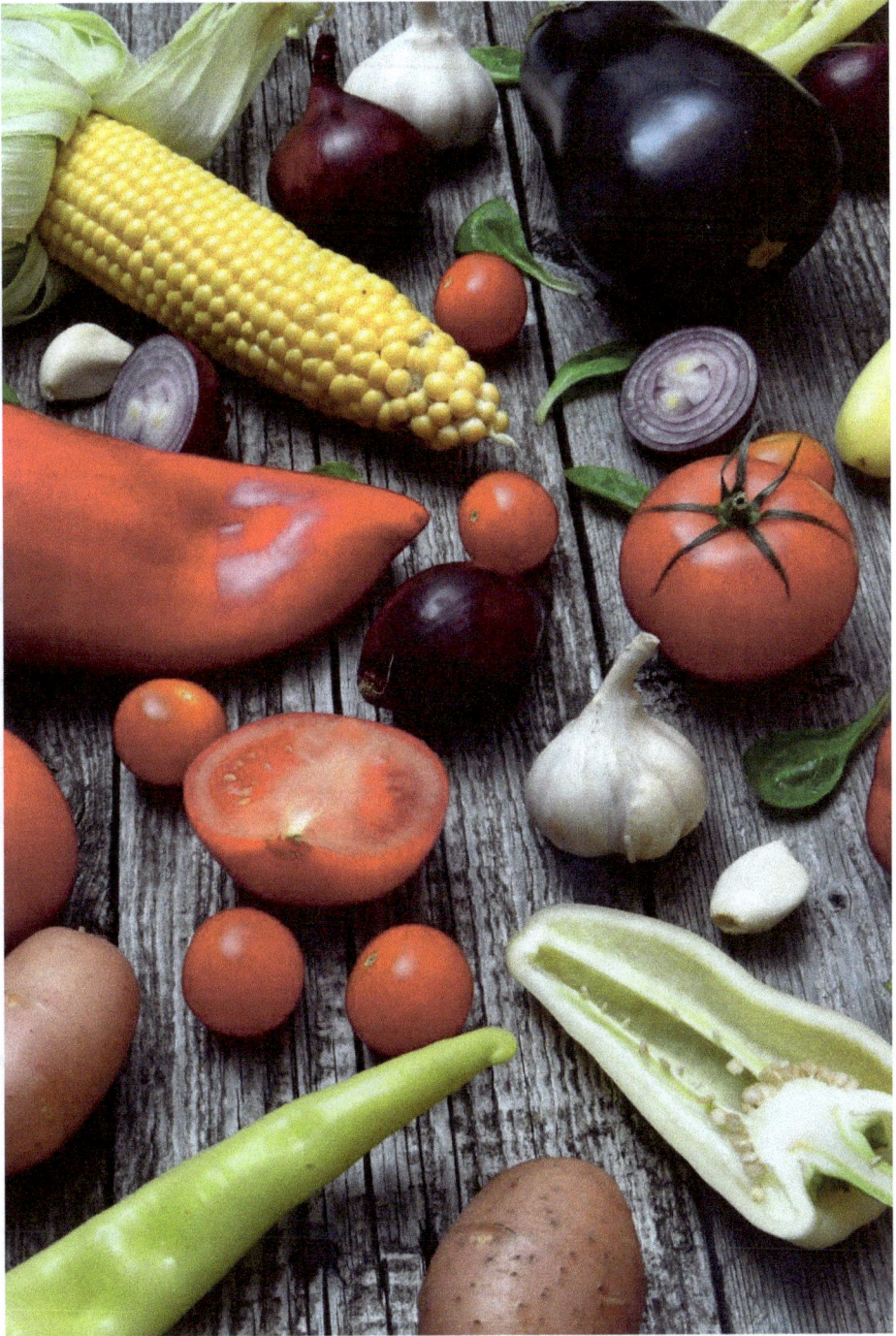

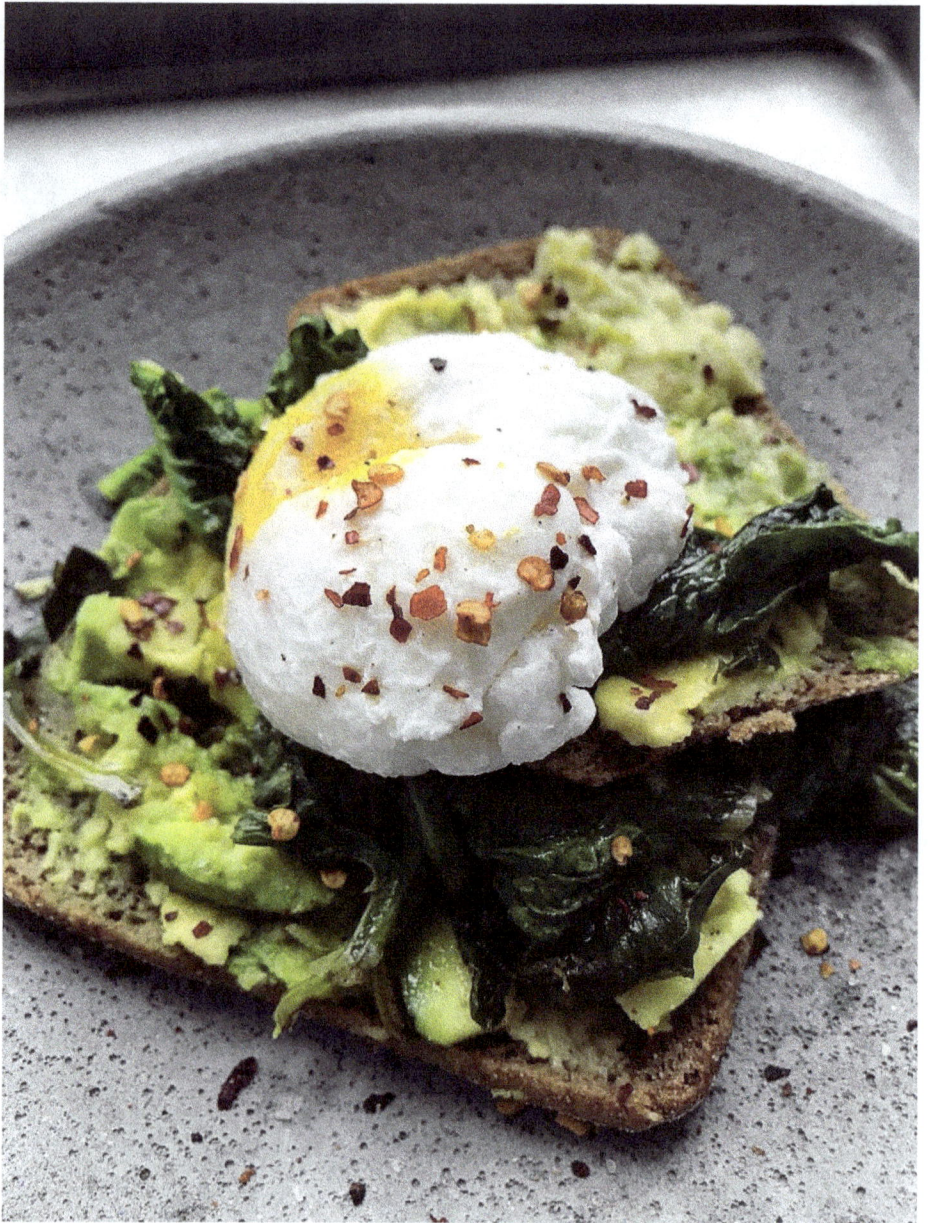

Glazed Beets

Preparation Time: 10 minutes Cooking Time: 50 minutes
Servings: 3

Ingredients

3 pounds beetroots, peeled and cut into medium chunks
4 tablespoons maple syrup 1 tablespoon olive oil

Directions:

Rub beets with the oil, add maple syrup, toss, introduce
in your Air Fryer and cook at 350 ° F for 40 minutes.
Divide between plates and serve as a side dish.

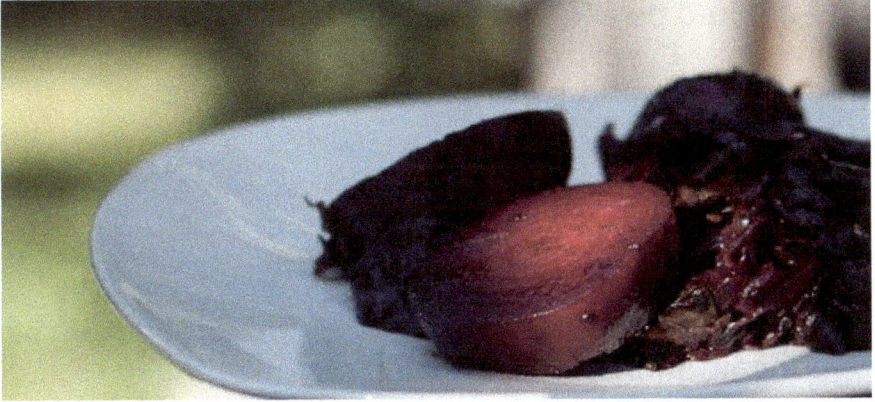

Easy Peppers Side Dish

Preparation Time: 10 minutes Cooking Time: 25 minutes
Servings: 1

Ingredients

12 colored bell peppers, seedless and sliced 1 tablespoon
olive oil 1 yellow onion, sliced ½ teaspoon smoked
paprika Salt and black pepper to the taste

Directions:

Put the oil in a pan that fits your Air Fryer, add bell
peppers, paprika and onion, toss, introduce the pan in
your Air Fryer and cook at 320 ° F for 25 minutes. Season
with salt and pepper to the taste, divide between plates
and serve as a side dish.

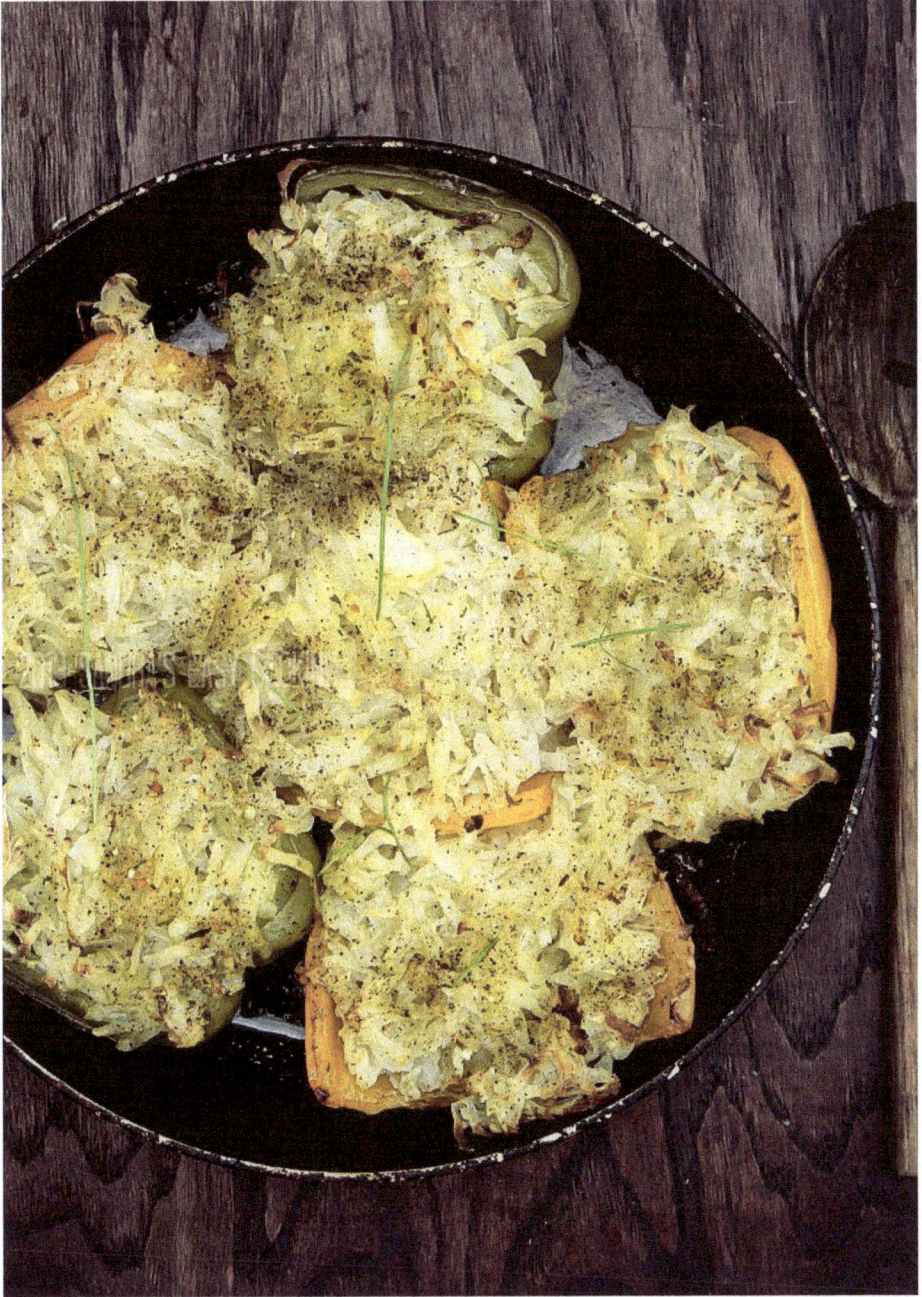

Tomatoes And Basil Mix

Preparation Time: 10 minutes Cooking Time: 14 minutes Servings: 4

Ingredients

1 bunch basil, chopped 3 garlic clove, minced A drizzle of olive oil Salt and black pepper to the taste 2 cups cherry tomatoes, halved

Directions:

In a pan that fits your Air Fryer, combine tomatoes with garlic, salt, pepper, basil and oil, toss, introduce in your Air Fryer and cook at 320 ° F for 12 minutes. Divide between plates and serve as a side dish.

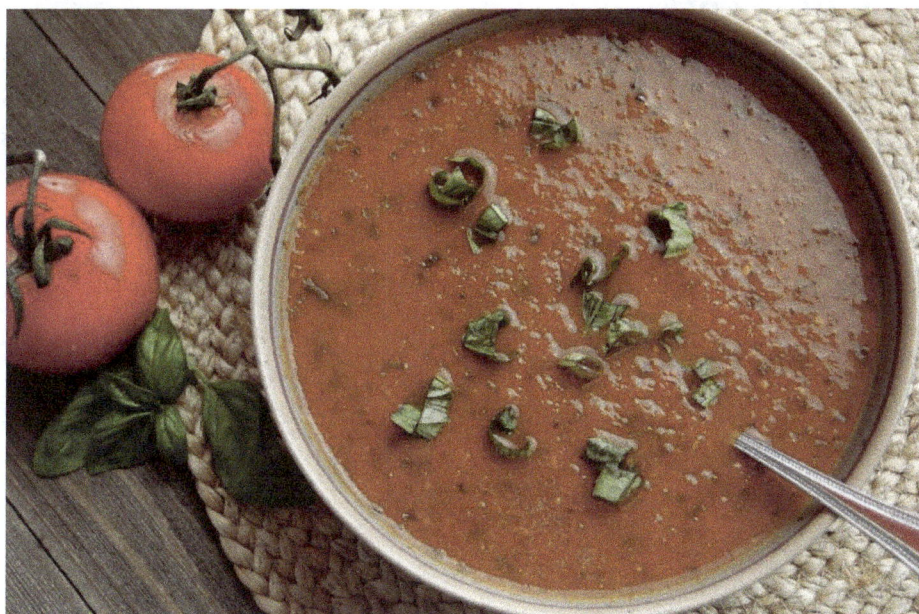

Red Potatoes And Green Beans

Preparation Time: 10 minutes Cooking Time: 15 minutes
Servings: 4

Ingredients

1 pound red potatoes, cut into wedges 1 pound green
beans 2 garlic cloves, minced 2 tablespoons olive oil Salt
and black pepper to the taste ½ teaspoon oregano, dried

Directions:

In a pan that fits your Air Fryer, combine potatoes with
green beans, garlic, oil, salt, pepper and oregano, toss,
introduce in your Air Fryer and cook at 380 ° F for 15
minutes. Divide between plates and serve as a side dish.

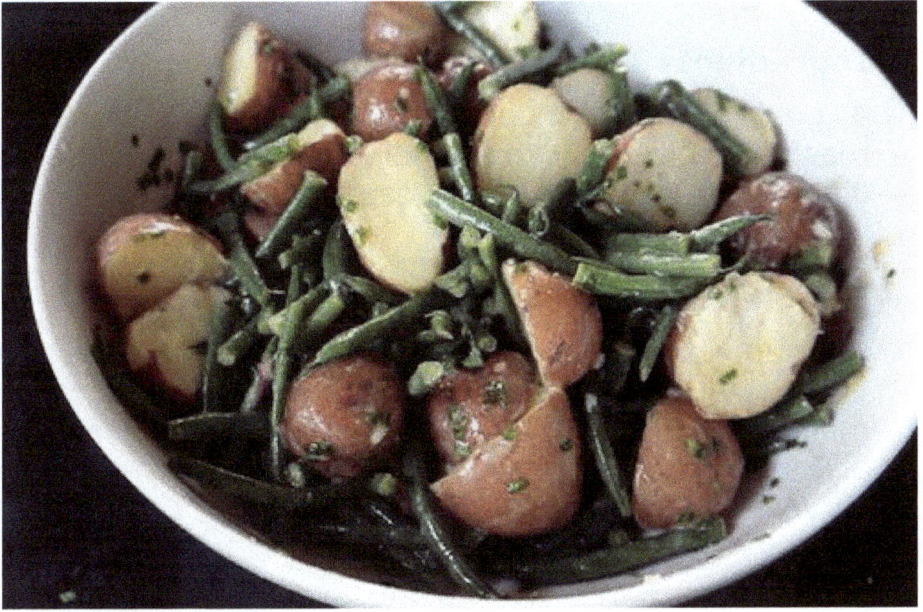

Gold Potatoes and Bell Pepper Mix

Preparation Time: 10 minutes Cooking Time: 25 minutes
Servings: 4

Ingredients

4 gold potatoes, cubed 1 yellow onion, chopped 2
teaspoons olive oil 1 green bell pepper, chopped Salt and
black pepper to the taste ½ teaspoon thyme, dried

Directions:

Heat up your Air Fryer at 350 ° F, add oil, heat it up, add
onion, bell pepper, salt and pepper, stir and cook for 5
minutes. Add potatoes and thyme, stir, cover and cook
at 360 °F for 20 minutes. Divide between plates and
serve as a side dish.

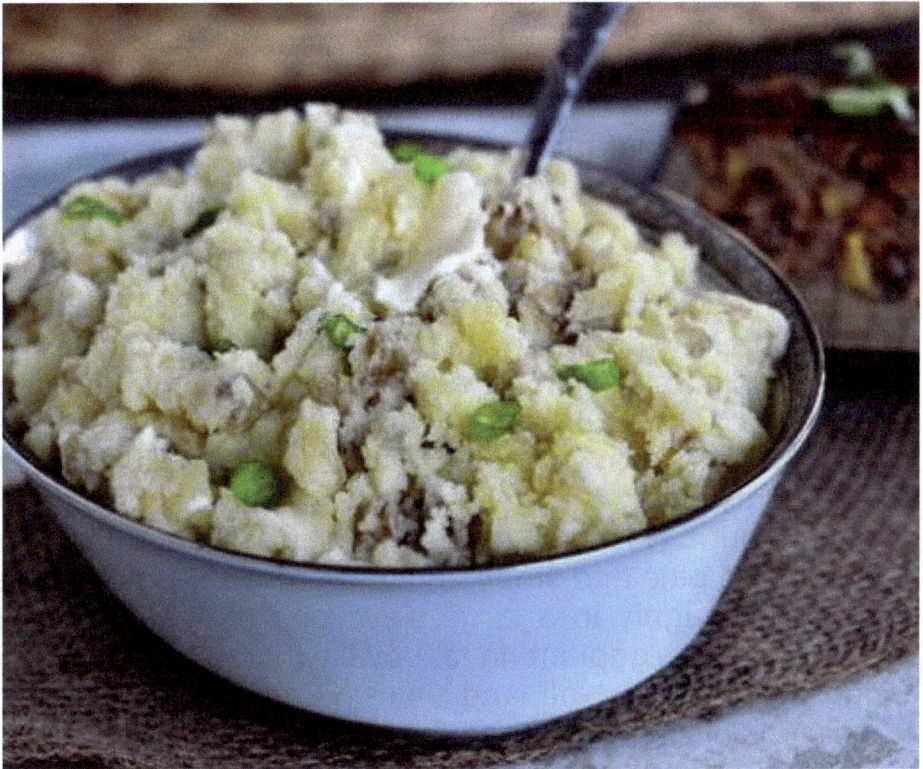

Eggplant Salad

Preparation time: 10 minutes Cooking time: 50 minutes
Servings: 3

Ingredients:

2 lbs. firm young eggplant 2½ Tbs. brown sugar 2 Tbs.
onion, minced 2 cloves garlic, minced 1 Tbs. olive oil 2
Tbs. cider vinegar 2 generous tsp. grated fresh ginger 2
tsp. fresh lemon juice

Directions:

Prick the eggplants in several places with a fork and roast
them in a 400 degree oven until they are quite soft. When
the eggplants are cool enough to handle, cut them in half
and scrape the pulp carefully out of the skin. If the seeds
are dark brown and starting to separate from the
eggplant, plant, they will be bitter and must be removed
(meaning it wasn't quite young or fresh enough). If the
seeds are pale and small, leave them. Drain the eggplant
pulp thoroughly in a large sieve and mince it. Combine
the minced eggplant in a bowl with all the remaining
ingredients, mix well, and chill several hours. Serve small
portions of the chilled eggplant on lettuce leaves as a first
course, or with unsalted crackers as a dip.

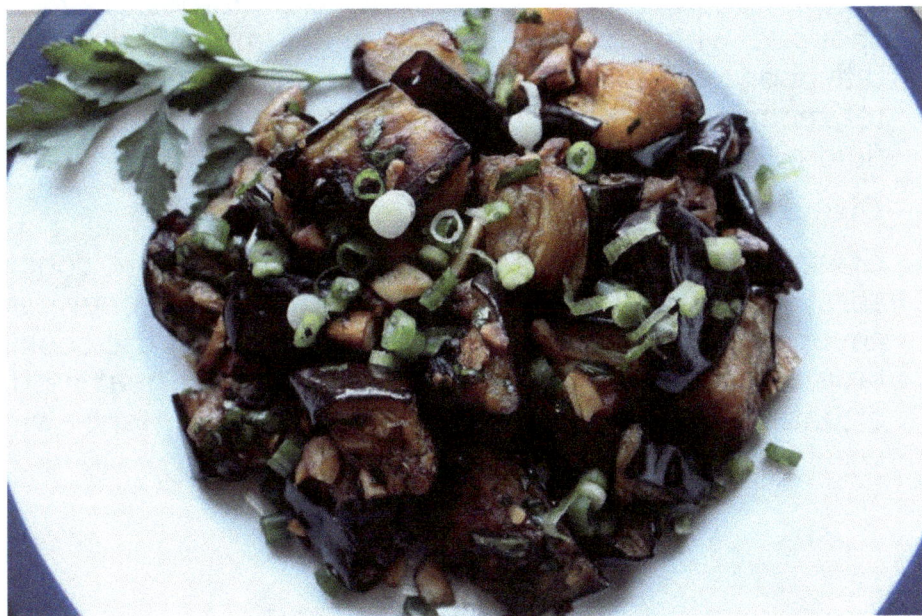

Savory Spanish Rice

Servings: 10 Preparation time: 3 hours and 10 minutes

Ingredients:

1 cup of long grain rice, uncooked 1/2 cup of chopped green bell pepper 14 ounce of diced tomatoes 1/2 cup of chopped white onion 1 teaspoon of minced garlic 1/2 teaspoon of salt 1 teaspoon of red chili powder 1 teaspoon of ground cumin 4-ounce of tomato puree 8 fluid ounce of water

Directions:

Grease a 6-quarts slow cooker with a non-stick cooking spray and add all the ingredients into it. Stir properly and cover the top. Plug in the slow cooker; adjust the cooking time to 5 hours and let it cook on the high heat setting or until the rice absorbs all the liquid. Serve right away.

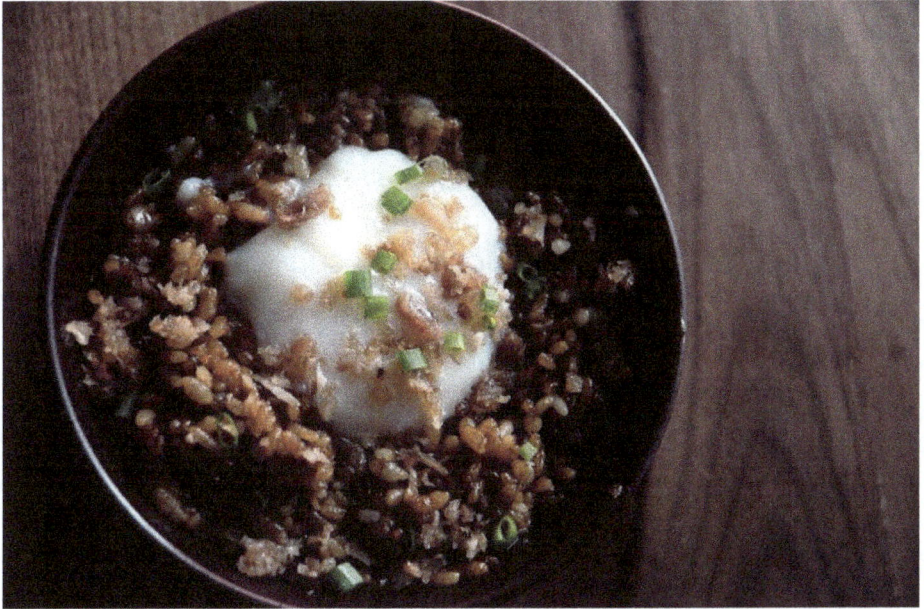

Tastiest Barbecued Tofu and Vegetables

Servings: 4 Preparation time: 4 hours 15 minutes

Ingredients:

14-ounce of extra-firm tofu, pressed and drained 2 medium-sized zucchini, steamed and diced 1/2 large green bell pepper, cored and cubed 3 stalks of broccoli stalks 8 ounce of sliced water chestnuts 1 small white onion, peeled and minced 1 1/2 teaspoon of minced garlic 2 teaspoons of minced ginger 1 1/2 teaspoon of salt 1/8 teaspoon of ground black pepper 1/4 teaspoon of crushed red pepper 1/4 teaspoon of five spice powder 2 teaspoons of molasses 1 tablespoon of whole-grain mustard 1/4 teaspoon of vegan Worcestershire sauce 8 ounces of tomato sauce 1/4 cup of hoisin sauce 1 tablespoon of soy sauce 2 tablespoons of apple cider vinegar 2 tablespoons of water

Directions:

Take a 6-quarts slow cooker, grease it with a non-stick cooking spray and set it aside until it is required. Place a medium-sized non-stick skillet pan over an average heat, add the oil and let it heat. Cut the tofu into 1/2 inch pieces and add it to the skillet pan in a single layer. Cook for 3 minutes per sides and then transfer it to the prepared slow cooker. When the tofu turns brown, place it into the pan, add the onion, garlic, ginger and cook for 3 to 5 minutes or until the onions are softened. Add the remaining ingredients into the pan except for the vegetables which are the broccoli stalks, zucchini, bell pepper and water chestnuts. Stir until it mixes properly and cook for 2 minutes or until the mixture starts bubbling. Transfer this mixture into the slow cooker and stir properly. Cover the top, plug in the slow cooker; adjust the cooking time to 3 hours and let it cook on the high heat setting or until it is cooked thoroughly. In the meantime, trim the broccoli stalks and cut it into 1/4 inch pieces. When the tofu is cooked thoroughly, put it into the slow cooker; add the broccoli stalks and the remaining vegetables. Stir until it mixes properly and then return the top to cover it. Continue cooking for 1 hour at the high heat setting or until the vegetables are tender. Serve right away with rice.

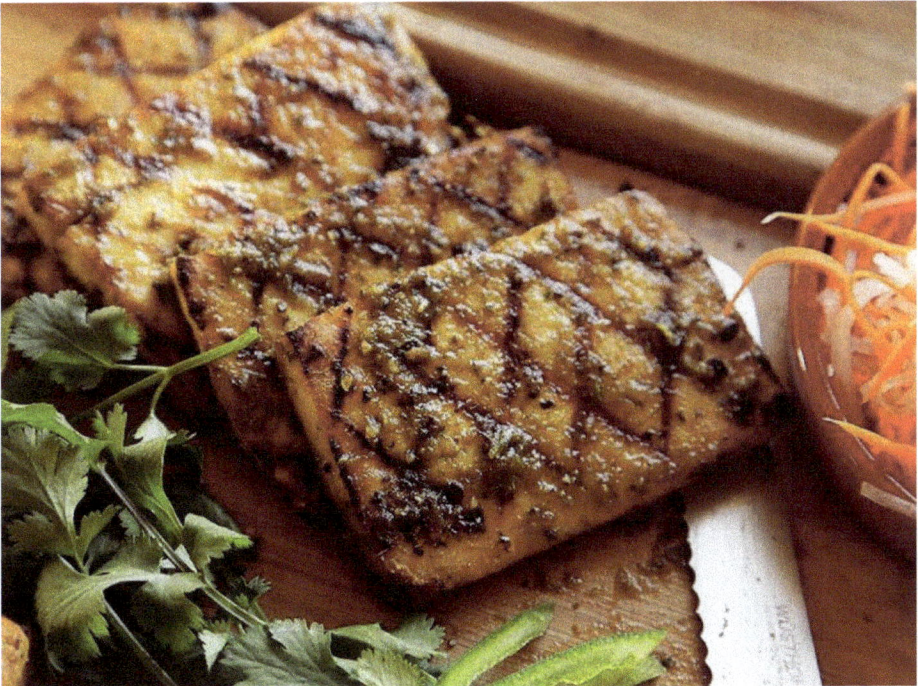

Super tasty Vegetarian Chili

Servings: 6 Preparation time: 2 hours and 10 minutes

Ingredients:

16-ounce of vegetarian baked beans 16 ounce of cooked chickpeas 16 ounce of cooked kidney beans 15 ounce of cooked corn 1 medium-sized green bell pepper, cored and chopped 2 stalks of celery, peeled and chopped 12 ounce of chopped tomatoes 1 medium-sized white onion, peeled and chopped 1 teaspoon of minced garlic 1 teaspoon of salt 1 tablespoon of red chili powder 1 tablespoon of dried oregano 1 tablespoon of dried basil 1 tablespoon of dried parsley 18-ounce of black bean soup 4-ounce of tomato puree

Directions:

Take a 6-quarts slow cooker, grease it with a non-stick cooking spray and place all the ingredients into it. Stir properly and cover the top. Plug in the slow cooker; adjust the cooking time to 2 hours and let it cook on the high heat setting or until it is cooked thoroughly. Serve right away.

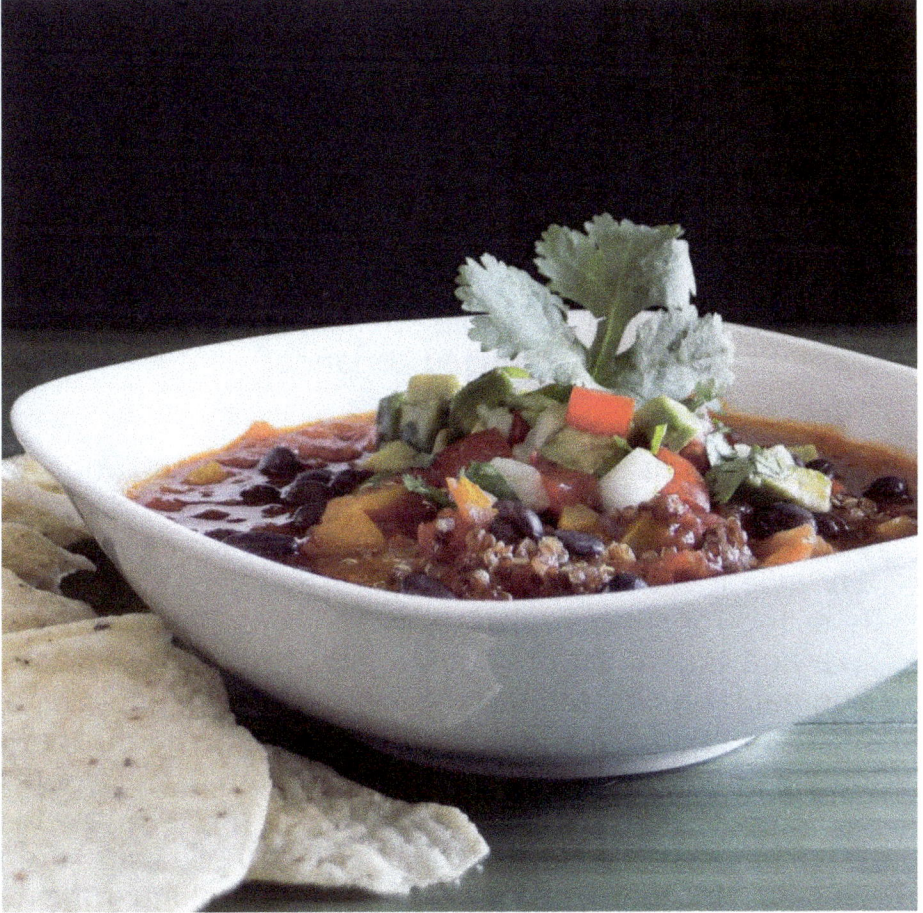

Comforting Chickpea Tagine

Servings: 6 Preparation time: 4 hours and 15 minutes

Ingredients:

14 ounce of cooked chickpeas 12 dried apricots 1 red bell pepper, cored and sliced 1 small butternut squash, peeled, cored and chopped 2 zucchini, stemmed and chopped 1 medium-sized white onion, peeled and chopped 1 teaspoon of minced garlic 1 teaspoon of ground ginger 1 1/2 teaspoon of salt 1 teaspoon of ground black pepper 1 teaspoon of ground cumin 2 teaspoon of paprika 1 teaspoon of harissa paste 2 teaspoon of honey 2 tablespoons of olive oil 1 pound of passata 1/4 cup of chopped coriander

Directions:

Take a 6-quarts slow cooker, grease it with a non-stick cooking spray and place the chickpeas, apricots, bell pepper, butternut squash, zucchini and onion into it. Sprinkle it with salt, black pepper and set it aside until it is called for. Place a large non-stick skillet pan over an average temperature of heat; add the oil, garlic, cumin and paprika. Stir properly and cook for 1 minutes or until it starts producing fragrance. Then pour in the harissa paste, honey, passata and boil the mixture. When the mixture is done boiling, pour this mixture over the vegetables in the slow cooker and cover it with the lid. Plug in the slow cooker; adjust the cooking time to 4 hours and let it cook on the high heat setting or until the vegetables gets tender. When done, add the seasoning, garnish it with the coriander and serve right away.

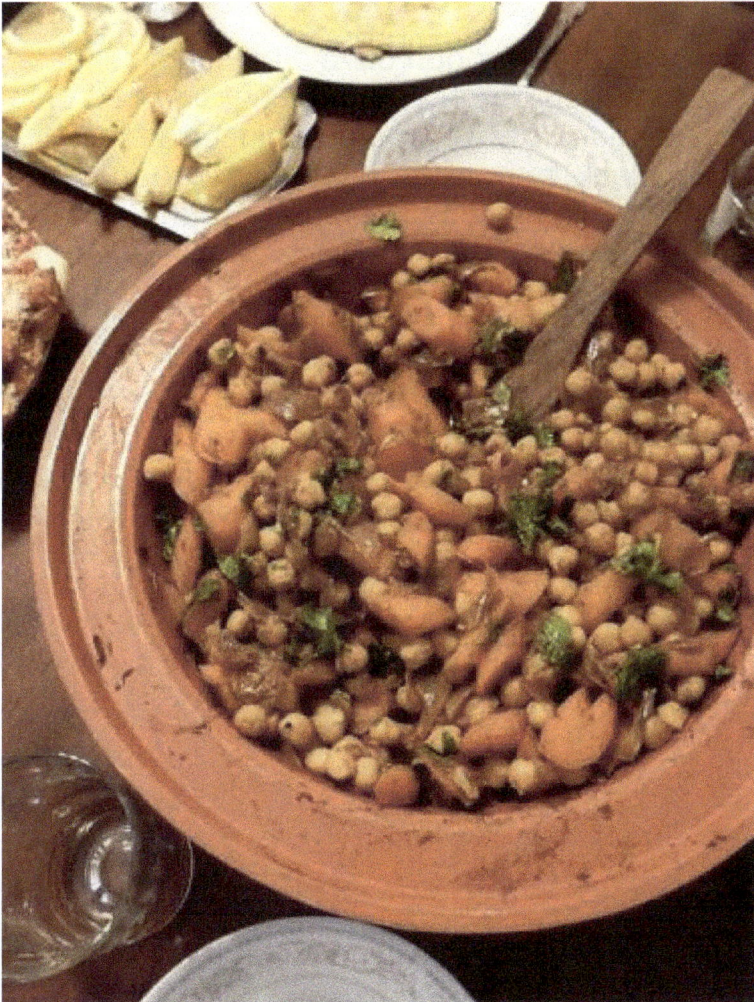

Falafel

Preparation time: 10 minutes Cooking time: 30 minutes
Servings: 4

Ingredients:

¼ cup and 1 tablespoon olive oil 1 cup chickpeas, cooked
½ cup chopped parsley ½ cup chopped red onion ½ cup
chopped cilantro 2 teaspoons minced garlic ½ teaspoon
ground black pepper ¼ teaspoon ground cinnamon 1
teaspoon of sea salt ½ teaspoon ground cumin

Directions:

Place all the ingredients in a food processor, reserving ¼
cup oil, and pulse until smooth. Shape the mixture into
small patties, place them on a rimmed baking sheet,
greased with remaining oil and bake for 30 minutes until
cooked and roasted on both sides, turning halfway
through. Serve straight away.

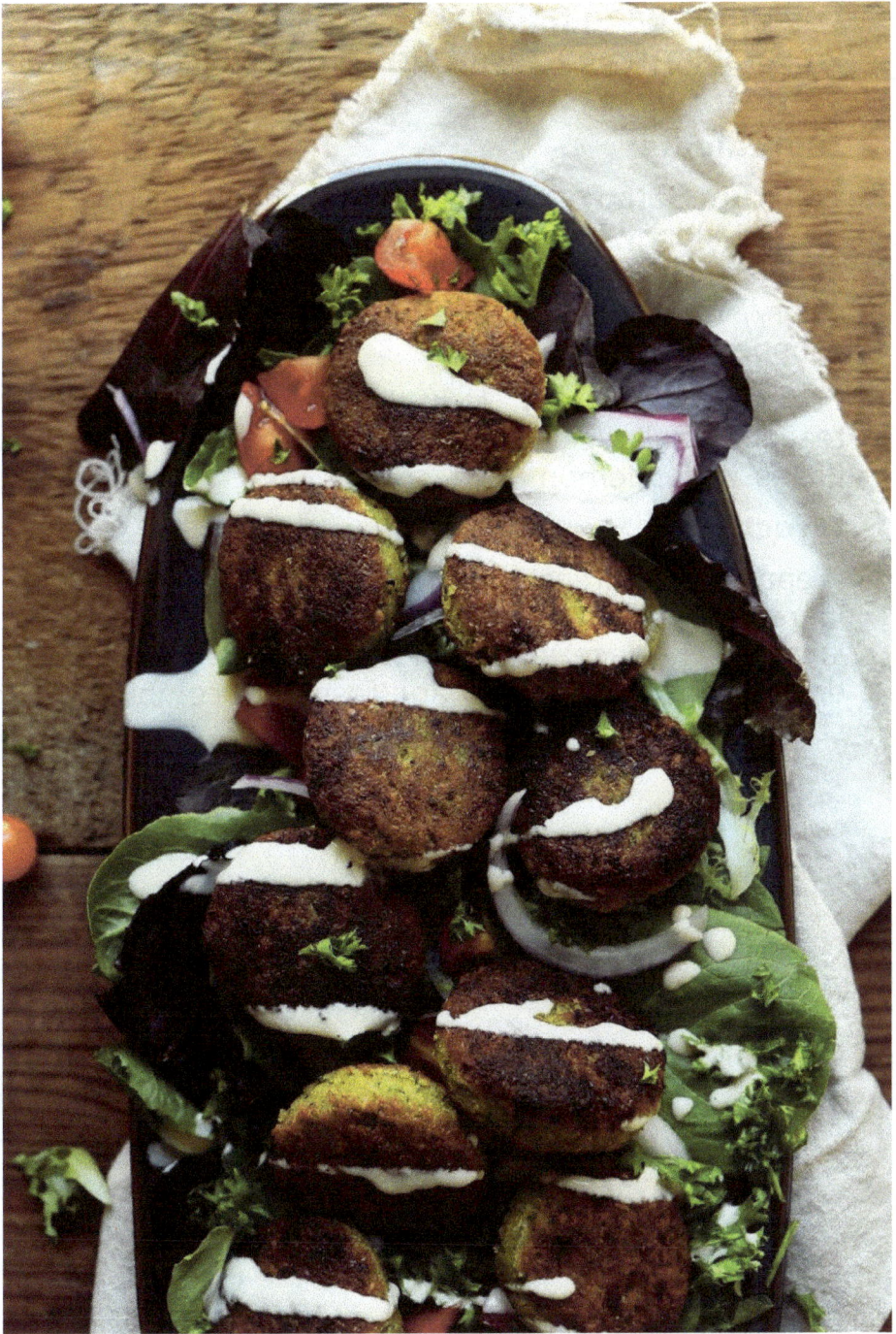

Lebanese Bean Salad

Preparation time: 10 minutes Cooking time: 0 minute Servings: 4

Ingredients:

For the Salad: 1 ½ cups cooked chickpeas 3 cups cooked kidney beans 1 small red onion, peeled, diced 1 medium cucumber, peeled, deseeded, diced 2 stalks celery, chopped ¾ cup chopped parsley 2 tablespoons chopped dill

For the Dressing: 1 ½ teaspoon minced garlic ¾ teaspoon salt ¼ cup olive oil 1/8 teaspoon red pepper flakes ¼ cup lemon juice

Directions:

Prepare the dressing and for this, place all of its ingredients in a bowl and whisk until combined. Take a large bowl, place all the ingredients for the salad in it, drizzle with the dressing and toss until combined. Serve straight away.

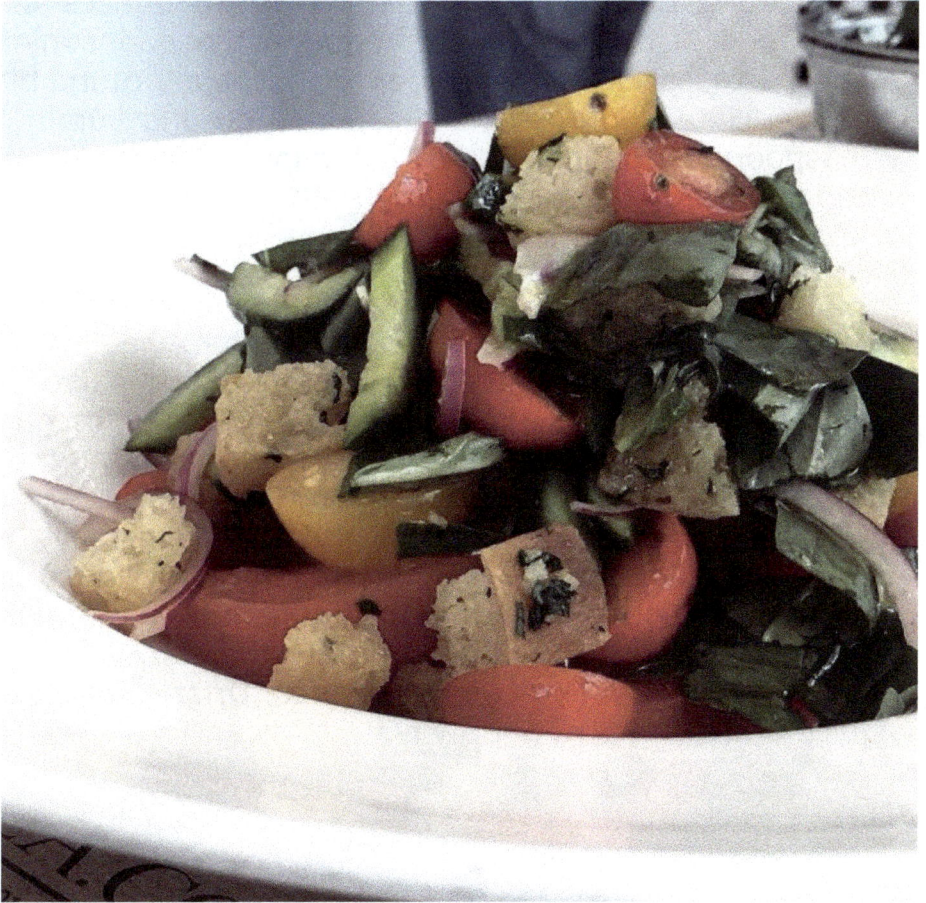

Lentil Soup

Preparation time: 10 minutes Cooking time: 50 minutes
Servings: 4

Ingredients:

1 cup green lentils 1 medium white onion, peeled,
chopped 1 cup chopped kale leaves 28 ounces diced
tomatoes 2 carrots, peeled, chopped 2 teaspoons minced
garlic 1 teaspoon curry powder ¼ teaspoon ground black
pepper 1 teaspoon salt 2 teaspoons ground cumin 1/8
teaspoon red pepper flakes ½ teaspoon dried thyme ¼
cup olive oil 4 cups vegetable broth 1 tablespoon lemon
juice 2 cups of water

Directions:

Take a large pot, place it over medium heat, add 1
tablespoon oil and when hot, add onion and carrot and
cook for 5 minutes until softened. Then stir in garlic,
curry powder, cumin and thyme, cook for 1 minute, then
stir in tomatoes and cook for 3 minutes. Add lentils, pour
in water and broth, season with black pepper, salt, and
red pepper and bring the mixture to a boil. Switch heat
to medium-low, simmer lentils for 30 minutes, then
puree half of the soup, return it into the pan, stir in kale
and cook for 5 minutes until softened. Drizzle with lemon
juice and serve straight away.

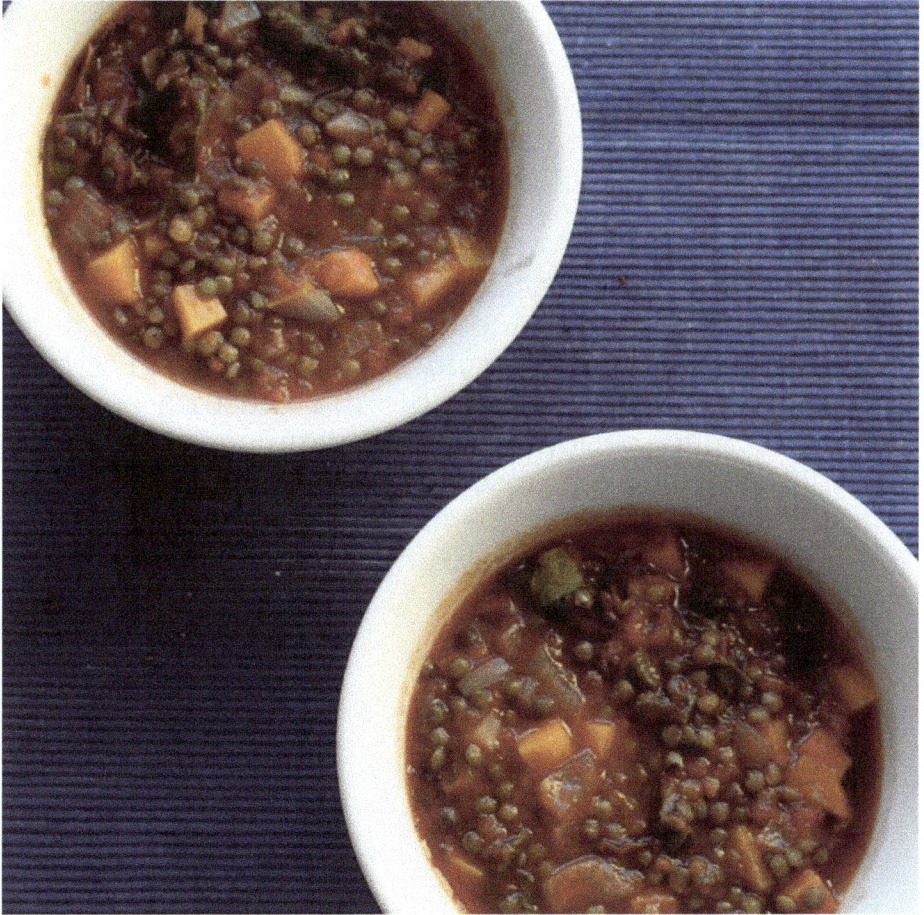

Quinoa and Black Beans

Preparation time: 10 minutes Cooking time: 35 minutes
Servings: 4

Ingredients:

3/4 cup quinoa 30 ounces cooked black beans 1 medium
white onion, peeled, chopped 1 ½ teaspoon minced garlic
1 cup frozen corn kernels ¼ teaspoon ground black
pepper 1/3 teaspoon salt 1 teaspoon ground cumin 1/4
teaspoon cayenne 1 teaspoon olive oil 1 1/2 cups
vegetable broth 1/2 cup chopped cilantro

Directions:

Take a saucepan, place it over medium heat, add oil and
when hot, add onion and garlic, and cook for 10 minutes
until softened. Add quinoa, pour in the broth, stir in all
the seasoning, then bring the mixture to a boil, switch
heat to medium-low level and simmer for 20 minutes
until the quinoa has absorbed all the liquid. Add corn, stir
until mixed, cook for 5 minutes until heated, and then
stir in beans until mixed. Garnish with cilantro and serve.

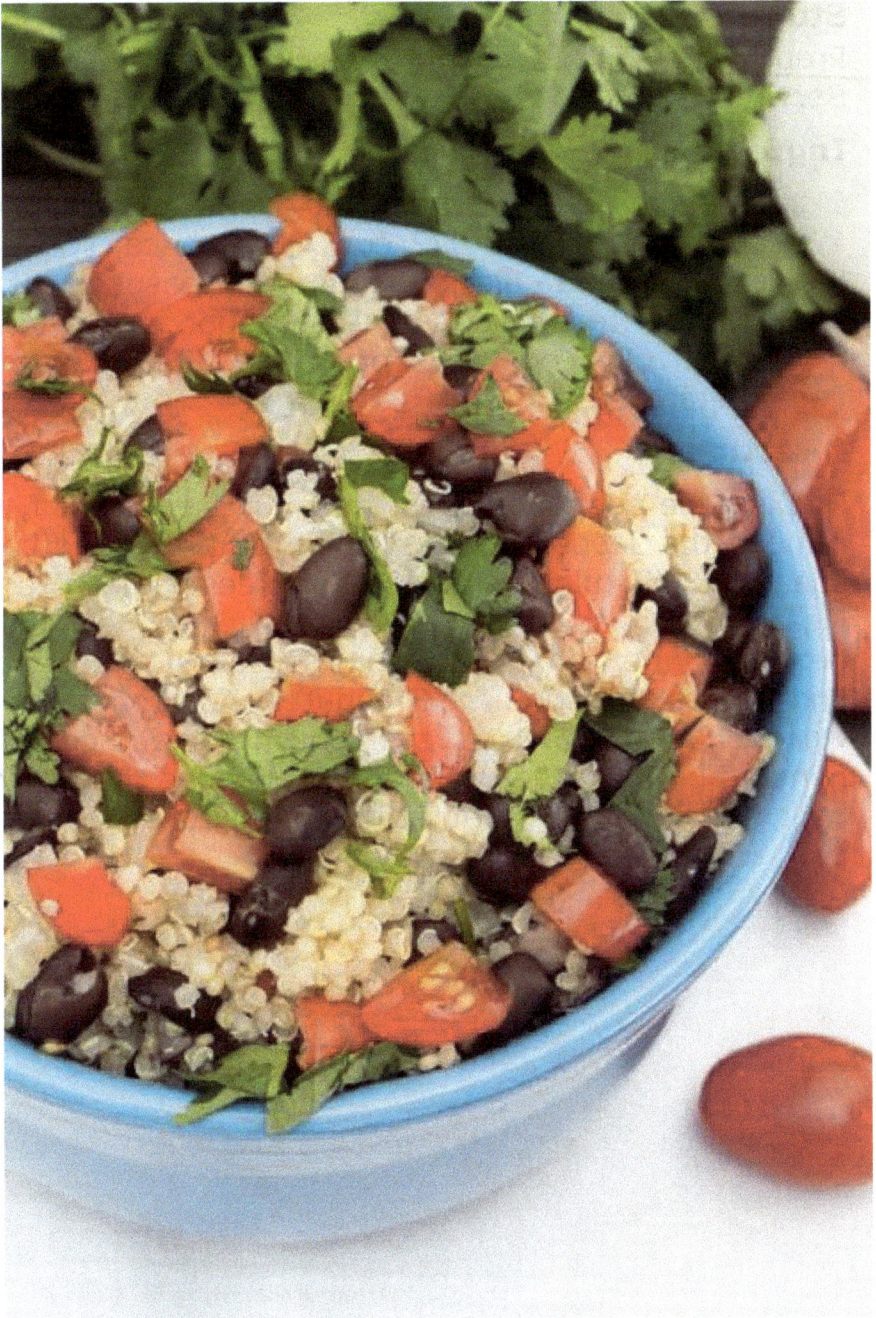

Stuffed Peppers

Preparation time: 10 minutes Cooking time: 20 minutes
Servings: 4

Ingredients:

2 green onions, sliced 2 green bell peppers, halved, cored
1 large tomato, diced 1/2 cup Arborio rice, cooked ¼
teaspoon ground black pepper 1 teaspoon Italian
seasoning 1 teaspoon salt 1 teaspoon dried basil 1
tablespoon olive oil 1 cup of water 1/2 cup crumbled
vegan feta cheese

Directions:

Prepare the peppers and for this, cut them in half, then
remove the seeds and roast them on a greased baking
sheet for 20 minutes at 400 degrees F until tender.
Meanwhile, heat oil in a skillet pan over medium-high
heat and when hot, add onion, season with seasonings
and herbs, and cook for 3 minutes. Add tomatoes, stir
well, cook for 5 minutes, then stir in rice and cook for 3
minutes until heated. When done, remove the pan from
heat, stir in cheese, and stuff the mixture into roasted
peppers. Serve straight away.

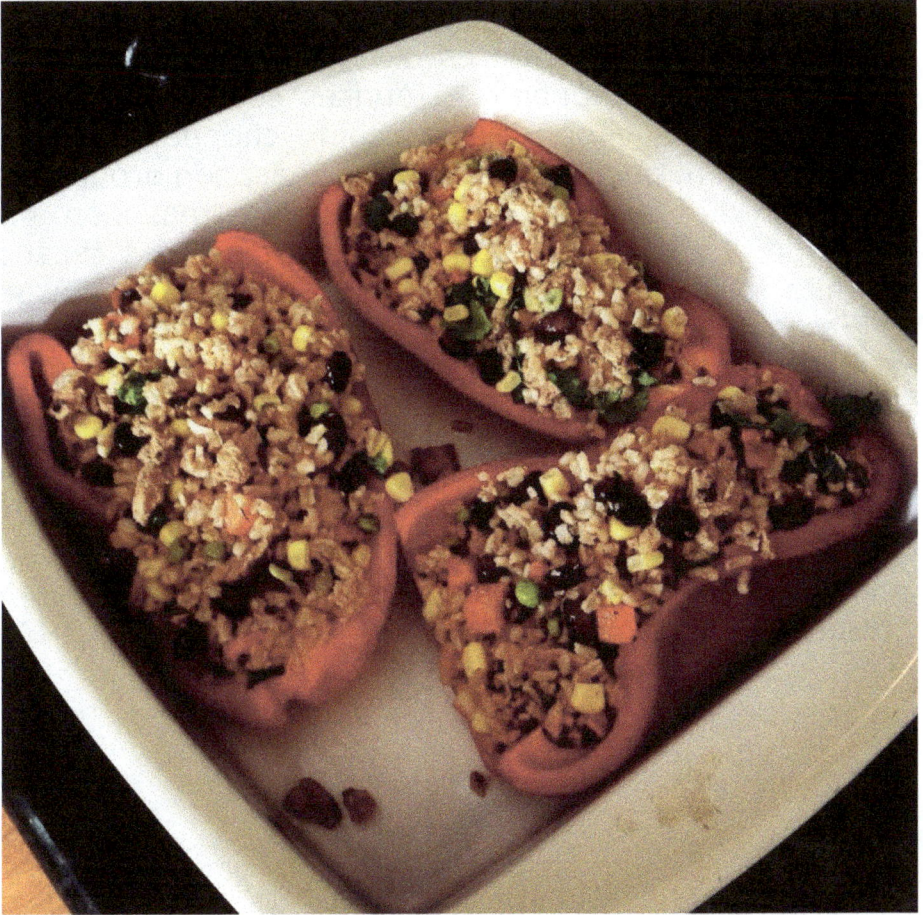

Vegetable Barley Soup

Preparation time: 5 minutes Cooking time: 15 minutes Servings: 8

Ingredients:

1 cup barley 14.5 ounces diced tomatoes with juice 2 large carrots, chopped 15 ounces cooked chickpeas 2 stalks celery, chopped 1 zucchini, chopped 1 medium white onion, peeled, chopped 1/2 teaspoon ground black pepper 1 teaspoon garlic powder 1 teaspoon curry powder 1 teaspoon salt 1 teaspoon paprika 1 teaspoon white sugar 1 teaspoon dried parsley 1 teaspoon Worcestershire sauce 3 bay leaves 2 quarts vegetable broth

Directions:

Place all the ingredients in a pot, stir until mixed, place it over medium-high heat and bring the mixture to a boil. Switch heat to medium level, simmer the soup for 90 minutes until cooked, and when done, remove bay leaf from it. Serve straight away.

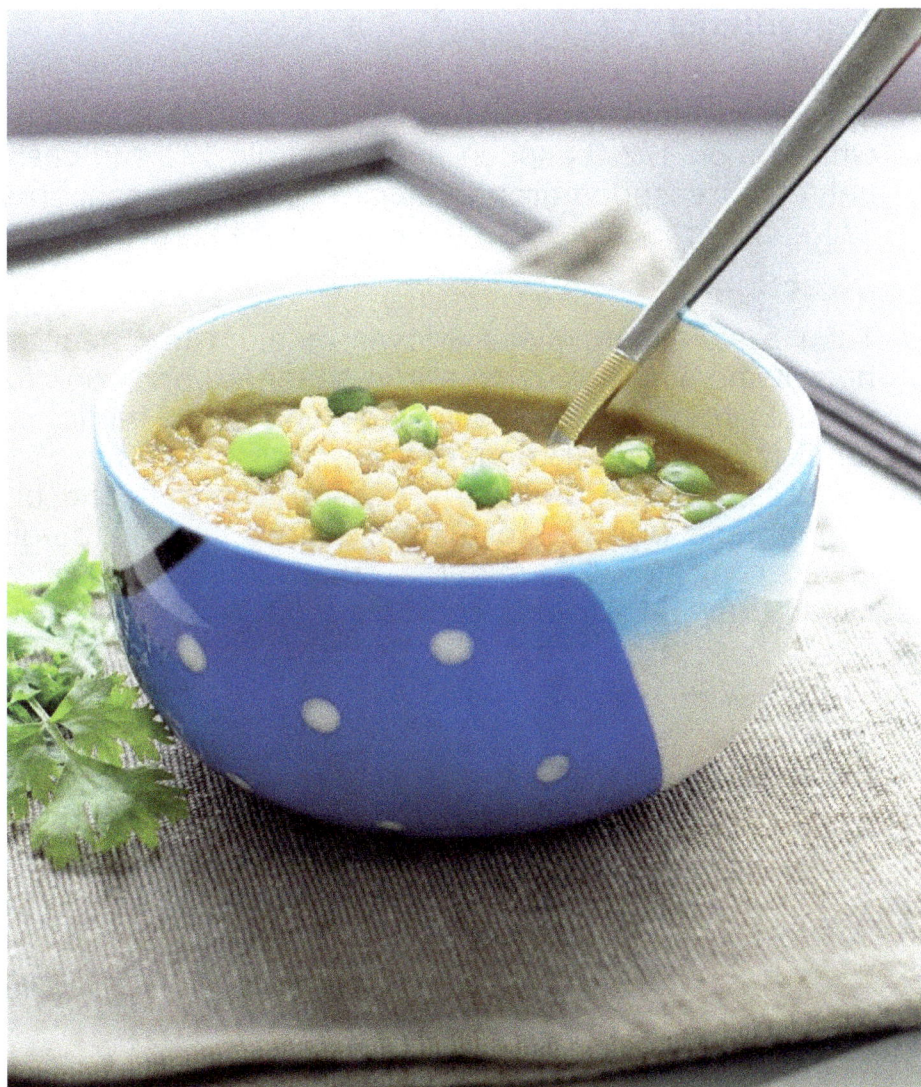

Asparagus Rice Pilaf

Preparation time: 10 minutes Cooking time: 35 minutes
Servings: 4

Ingredients:

1 1/4 cups rice 1/2 pound asparagus, diced, boiled 2 ounces spaghetti, whole-grain, broken 1/4 cup minced white onion 1/2 teaspoon minced garlic 1/2 cup cashew halves ¼ teaspoon ground black pepper ½ teaspoon salt 1/4 cup vegan butter 2 1/4 cups vegetable broth

Directions:

Take a saucepan, place it over medium-low heat, add butter and when it melts, stir in spaghetti and cook for 3 minutes until golden brown. Add onion and garlic, cook for 2 minutes until tender, then stir in rice, cook for 5 minutes, pour in the broth, season with salt and black pepper and bring it to a boil. Switch heat to medium level, cook for 20 minutes, then add cashews and asparagus and stir until combined. Serve straight away.

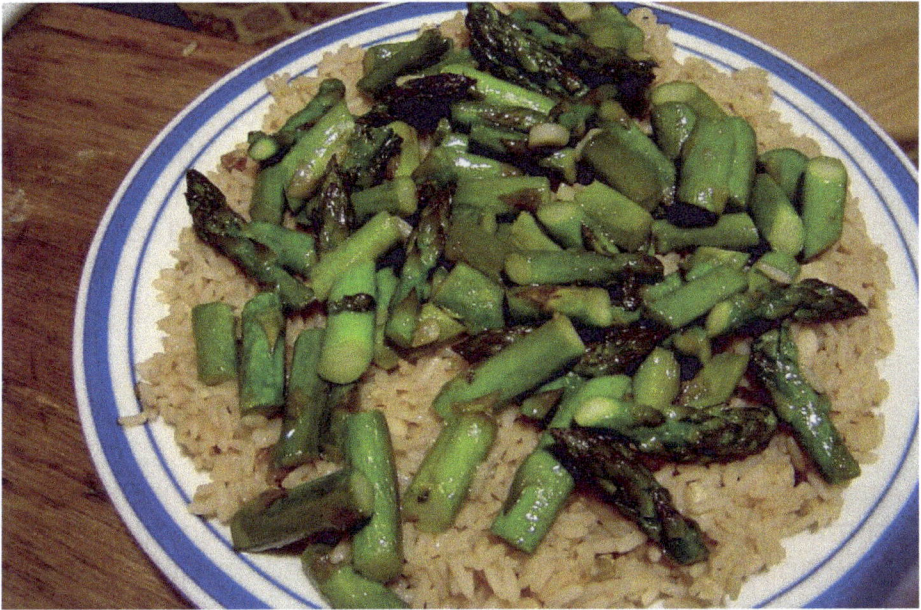

Quinoa and Black Bean Chili

Preparation time: 10 minutes Cooking time: 32 minutes Servings: 10

Ingredients:

1 cup quinoa, cooked 38 ounces cooked black beans 1 medium white onion, peeled, chopped 1 cup of frozen corn 1 green bell pepper, deseeded, chopped 1 zucchini, chopped 1 tablespoon minced chipotle peppers in adobo sauce 1 red bell pepper, deseeded, chopped 1 jalapeno pepper, deseeded, minced 28 ounces crushed tomatoes 2 teaspoons minced garlic 1/3 teaspoon ground black pepper ¾ teaspoon salt 1 teaspoon dried oregano 1 tablespoon red chili powder 1 tablespoon ground cumin 1 tablespoon olive oil 1/4 cup chopped cilantro

Directions:

Take a large pot, place it over medium heat, add oil and when hot, add onion and cook for 5 minutes. Then stir in garlic, cumin, and chili powder, cook for 1 minute, add remaining ingredients except for corn and quinoa, stir well and simmer for 20 minutes at medium-low heat until cooked. Then stir in corn and quinoa, cook for 5 minutes until hot and then top with cilantro. Serve straight away.

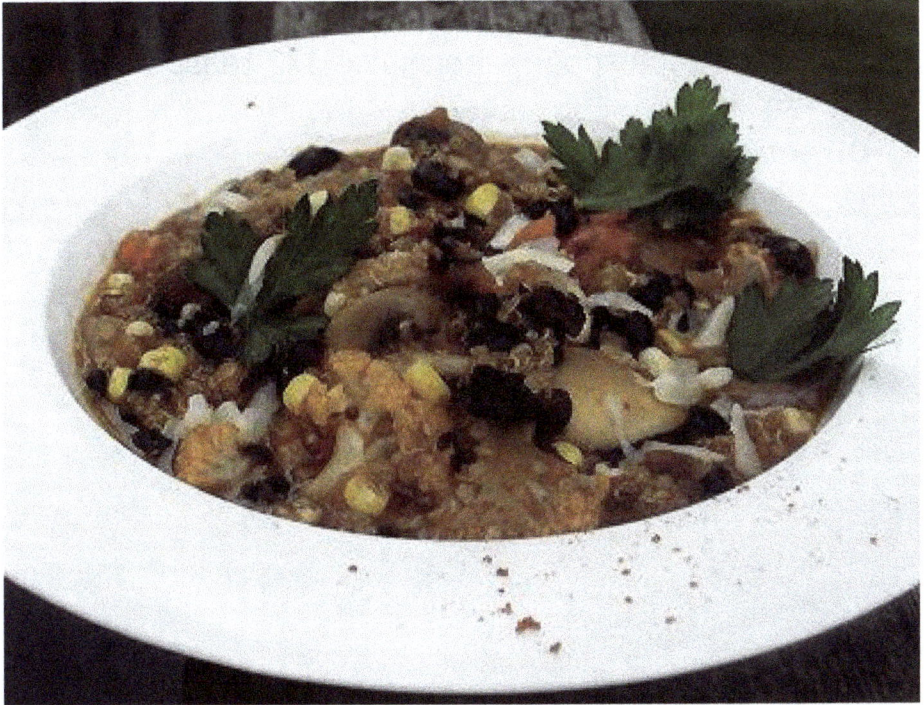

Quinoa with Chickpeas and Tomatoes

Preparation time: 10 minutes Cooking time: 0 minute
Servings: 6

Ingredients:

1 tomato, chopped 1 cup quinoa, cooked ½ teaspoon
minced garlic ¼ teaspoon ground black pepper ½
teaspoon salt 1/2 teaspoon ground cumin 4 teaspoons
olive oil 3 tablespoons lime juice 1/2 teaspoon chopped
parsley

Directions:

Take a large bowl, place all the ingredients in it, except
for the parsley, and stir until mixed. Garnish with parsley
and serve straight away.

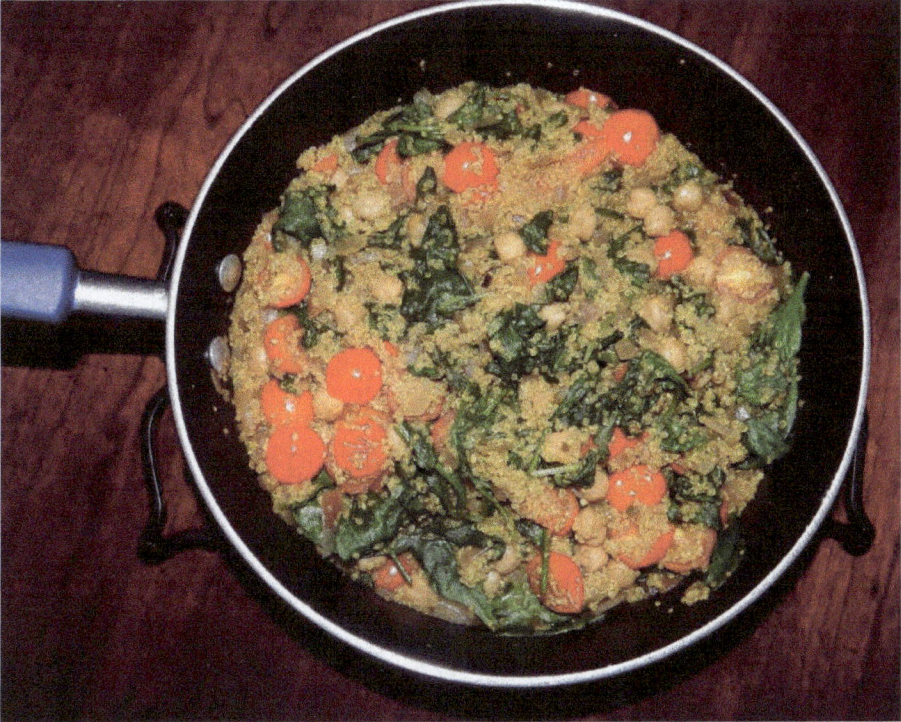

Zucchini Risotto

Preparation time: 10 minutes Cooking time: 30 minutes Servings: 6

Ingredients:

2 cups Arborio rice 10 sun-dried tomatoes, chopped 1 medium white onion, peeled, chopped 1 tablespoon chopped basil leaves 1/2 medium zucchini, sliced 1 teaspoon dried thyme 1/3 teaspoon ground black pepper 1 tablespoon vegan butter 6 tablespoons grated vegan Parmesan cheese 7 cups vegetable broth, hot

Directions: Take a large pot, place it over medium heat, add butter and when it melts, add onion and cook for 2 minutes. Stir in rice, cook for another 2 minutes until toasted, and then stir in broth, 1 cup at a time until absorbed completely and creamy mixture comes together. Then stir in remaining ingredients until combined, taste to adjust seasoning and serve

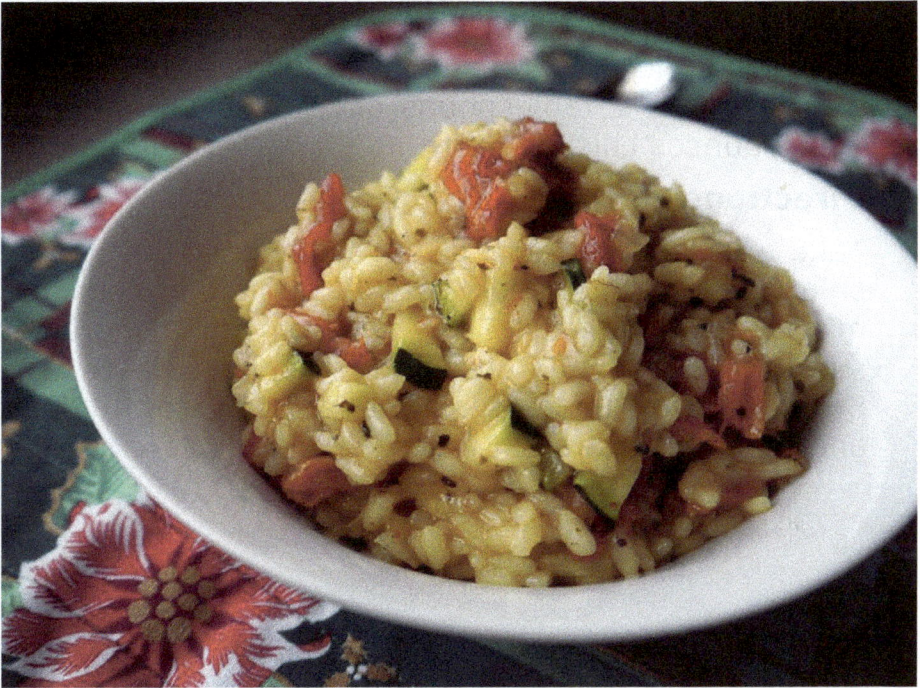

Tomato Barley Soup

Preparation time: 10 minutes Cooking time: 40 minutes Servings: 6

Ingredients:

1/4 cup barley 1 cup chopped celery 14.5 ounces peeled and diced tomatoes 1 cup chopped white onions 2 tomatoes, diced 1 cup chopped carrots 2 teaspoons minced garlic 1/8 teaspoon ground black pepper 1 teaspoon salt 2 tablespoons olive oil 2 1/2 cups water 10.75 ounces chicken broth

Directions:

Take a large saucepan, place it over medium heat, add onion, carrot, and celery, stir in garlic and cook for 10 minutes until tender. Then add remaining ingredients, stir until combined, and bring the mixture to a boil. Switch heat to the level, simmer the soup for 40 minutes and then serve straight away.

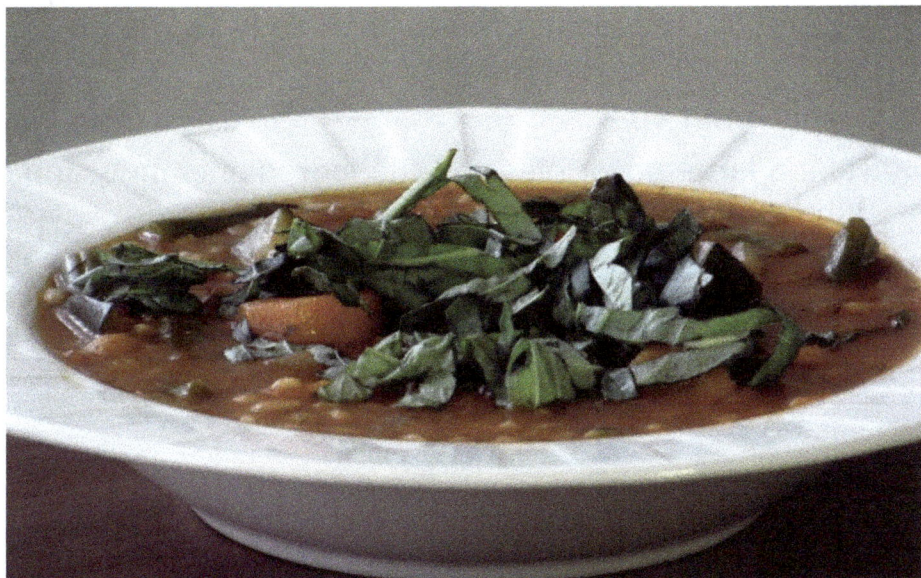

Lemony Quinoa

Preparation time: 10 minutes Cooking time: 0 minute Servings: 6

Ingredients:

1 cup quinoa, cooked 1/4 of medium red onion, peeled, chopped 1 bunch of parsley, chopped 2 stalks of celery, chopped ¼ teaspoon of sea salt 1/4 teaspoon cayenne pepper 1/2 teaspoon ground cumin 1/4 cup lemon juice 1/4 cup pine nuts, toasted

Directions:

Take a large bowl, place all the ingredients in it, and stir until combined. Serve straight away.

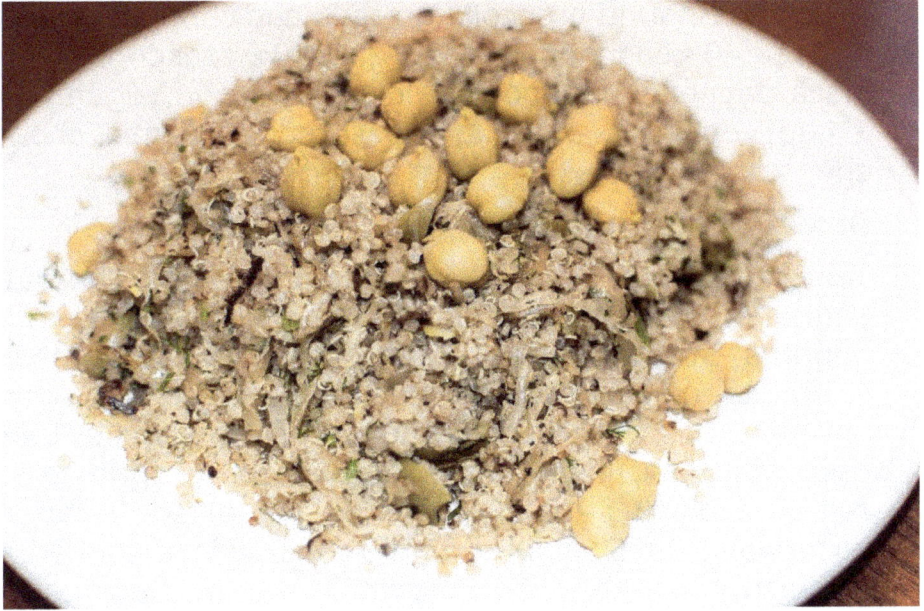

Brown Rice, Broccoli, and Walnut

Preparation time: 5 minutes Cooking time: 18 minutes Servings: 4

Ingredients:

1 cup of brown rice 1 medium white onion, peeled, chopped 1 pound broccoli florets ½ cup chopped walnuts, toasted ½ teaspoon minced garlic ⅛ teaspoon ground black pepper ½ teaspoon salt 1 tablespoon vegan butter 1 cup vegetable broth 1 cup shredded vegan cheddar cheese

Directions:

Take a saucepan, place it over medium heat, add butter and when it melts, add onion and garlic and cook for 3 minutes. Stir in rice, pour in the broth, bring the mixture to boil, then switch heat to medium-low level and simmer until rice has absorbed all the liquid. Meanwhile, take a casserole dish, place broccoli florets in it, sprinkle with salt and black pepper, cover with a plastic wrap and microwave for 5 minutes until tender. Place cooked rice in a dish, top with broccoli, sprinkle with nuts and cheese, and then serve.

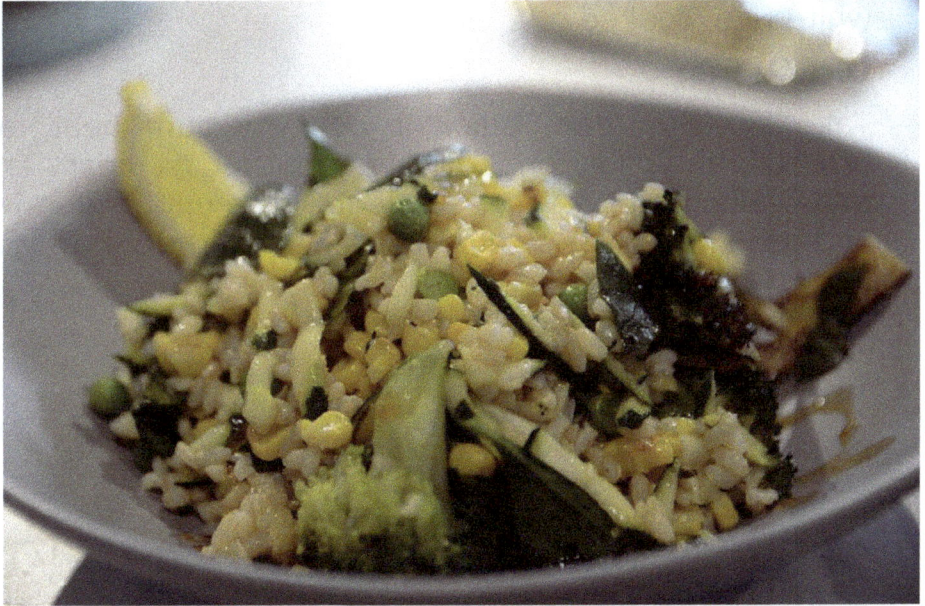

Broccoli and Rice Stir Fry

Preparation time: 5 minutes Cooking time: 10 minutes
Servings: 8

Ingredients:

16 ounces frozen broccoli florets, thawed 3 green onions, diced ½ teaspoon salt ¼ teaspoon ground black pepper 2 tablespoons soy sauce 1 tablespoon olive oil 1 ½ cups white rice, cooked

Directions:

Take a skillet pan, place it over medium heat, add broccoli, and cook for 5 minutes until tender-crisp. Then add scallion and other ingredients, toss until well mixed and cook for 2 minutes until hot. Serve straight away.

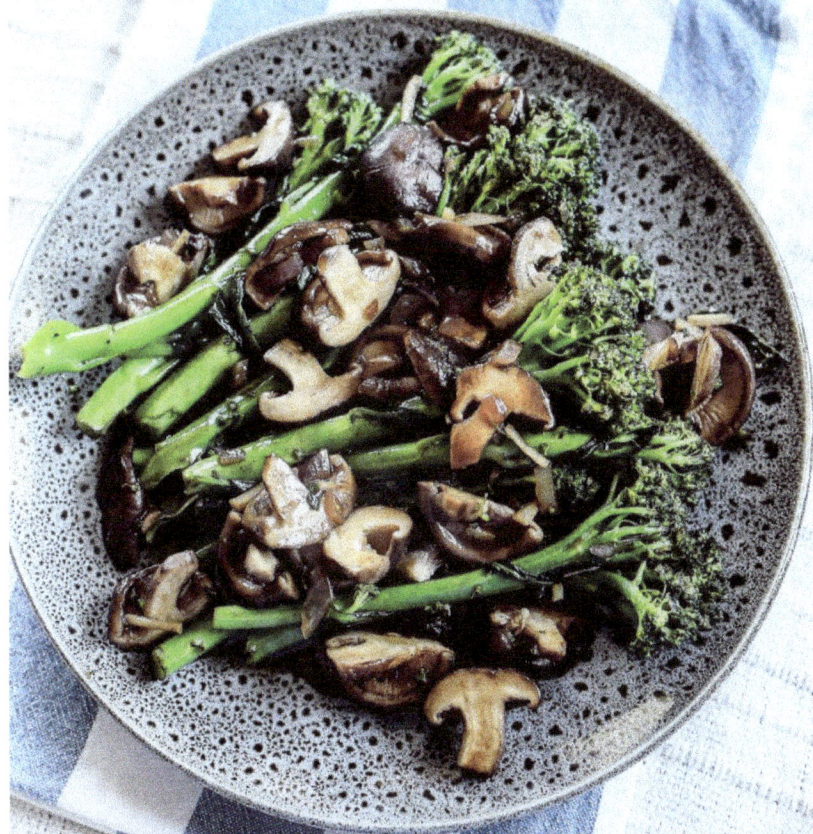

Coconut Rice

Preparation time: 10 minutes Cooking time: 25 minutes
Servings: 7

Ingredients:

2 1/2 cups white rice 1/8 teaspoon salt 40 ounces
coconut milk, unsweetened

Directions:

Take a large saucepan, place it over medium heat, add
all the ingredients in it and stir until mixed. Bring the
mixture to a boil, then switch heat to medium-low level
and simmer rice for 25 minutes until tender and all the
liquid is absorbed. Serve straight away.

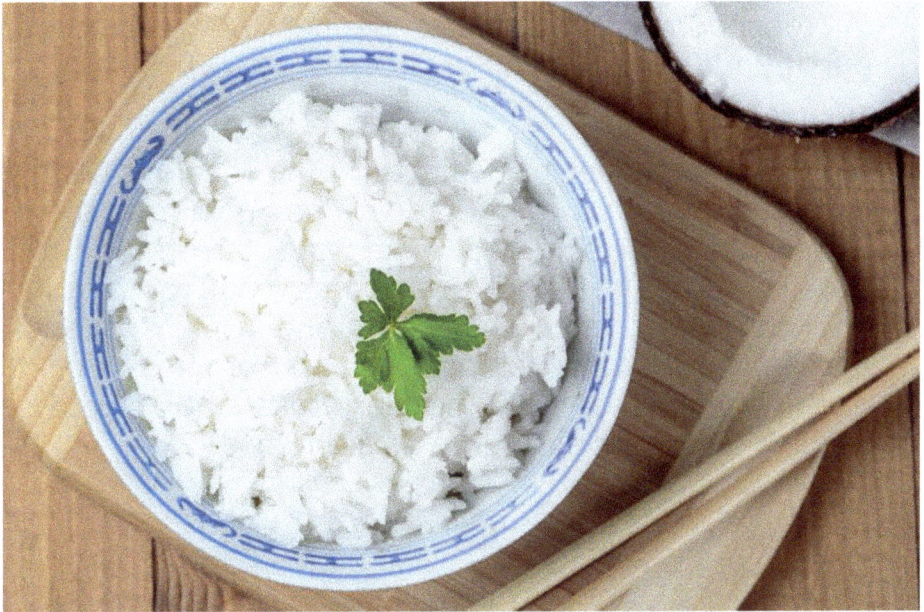

Brown Rice Pilaf

Preparation time: 5 minutes Cooking time: 25 minutes
Servings: 4

Ingredients:

1 cup cooked chickpeas 3/4 cup brown rice, cooked 1/4
cup chopped cashews 2 cups sliced mushrooms 2 carrots,
sliced ½ teaspoon minced garlic 1 1/2 cups chopped
white onion 3 tablespoons vegan butter ½ teaspoon salt
¼ teaspoon ground black pepper 1/4 cup chopped
parsley

Directions:

Take a large skillet pan, place it over medium heat, add
butter and when it melts, add onions and cook them for
5 minutes until softened. Then add carrots and garlic,
cook for 5 minutes, add mushrooms, cook for 10 minutes
until browned, add chickpeas and cook for another
minute. When done, remove the pan from heat, add nuts,
parsley, salt and black pepper, toss until mixed, and
garnish with parsley. Serve straight away.

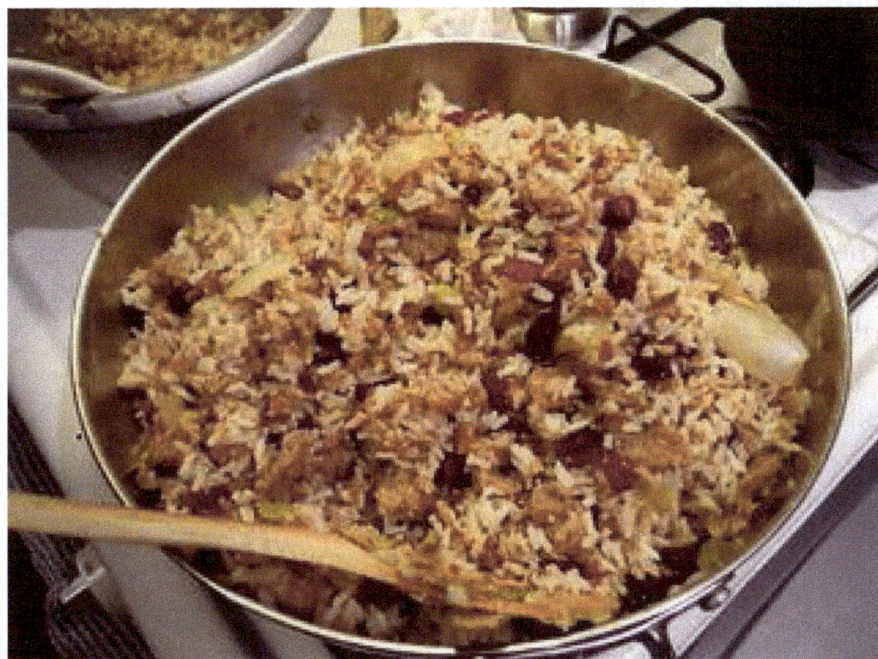

Vegan Curried Rice

Preparation time: 5 minutes Cooking time: 25 minutes Servings: 4

Ingredients:

1 cup white rice 1 tablespoon minced garlic 1 tablespoon ground curry powder 1/3 teaspoon ground black pepper 1 tablespoon red chili powder 1 tablespoon ground cumin 2 tablespoons olive oil 1 tablespoon soy sauce 1 cup vegetable broth

Directions: Take a saucepan, place it over low heat, add oil and when hot, add garlic and cook for 3 minutes. Then stir in all spices, cook for 1 minute until fragrant, pour in the broth, and switch heat to a high level. Stir in soy sauce, bring the mixture to boil, add rice, stir until mixed, then switch heat to the low level and simmer for 20 minutes until rice is tender and all the liquid has absorbed. Serve straight away.

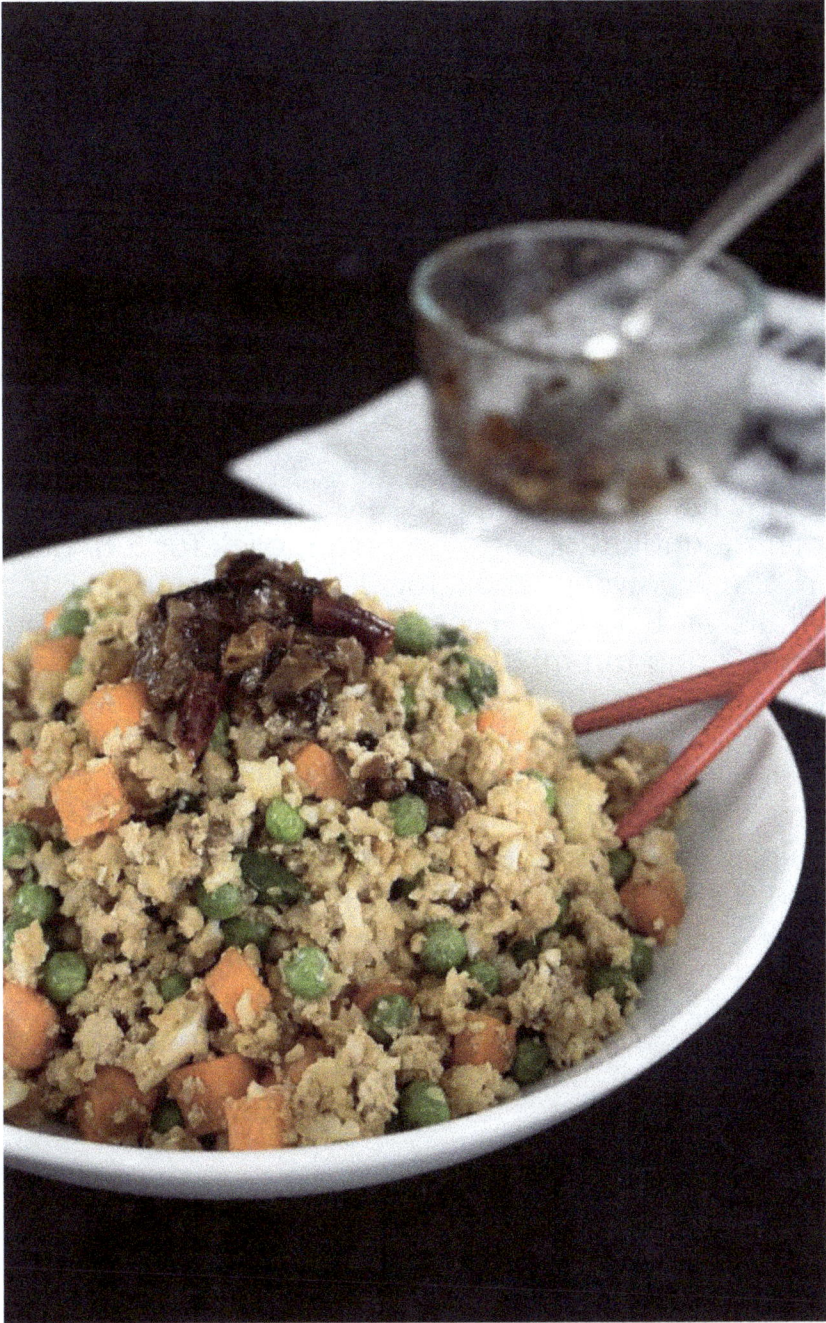

Coconut Curry Lentils

Preparation time: 10 minutes Cooking time: 40 minutes Servings: 4

Ingredients:

1 cup brown lentils 1 small white onion, peeled, chopped 1 teaspoon minced garlic 1 teaspoon grated ginger 3 cups baby spinach 1 tablespoon curry powder 2 tablespoons olive oil 13 ounces coconut milk, unsweetened 2 cups vegetable broth For Serving: 4 cups cooked rice 1/4 cup chopped cilantro

Directions: Place a large pot over medium heat, add oil and when hot, add ginger and garlic and cook for 1 minute until fragrant. Add onion, cook for 5 minutes, stir in curry powder, cook for 1 minute until toasted, add lentils and pour in broth. Switch heat to medium-high level, bring the mixture to a boil, then switch heat to the low level and simmer for 20 minutes until tender and all the liquid is absorbed. Pour in milk, stir until combined, turn heat to medium level, and simmer for 10 minutes until thickened. Then remove the pot from heat, stir in spinach, let it stand for 5 minutes until its leaves wilts and then top with cilantro. Serve lentils with rice.

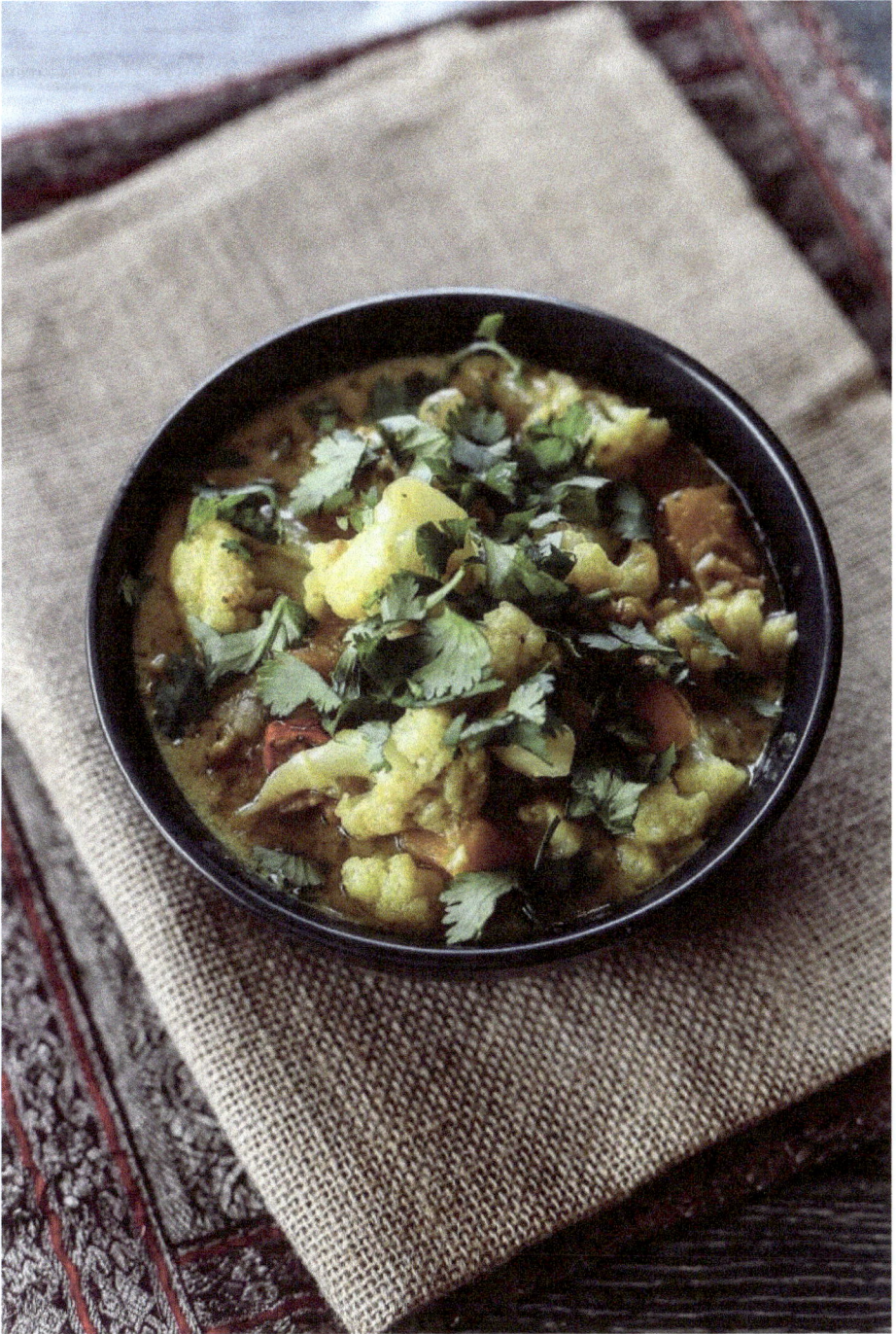

Chard Wraps With Millet

Preparation time: 25 minutes Cooking time: 0 minute Servings: 4

Ingredients:

1 carrot, cut into ribbons 1/2 cup millet, cooked 1/2 of a large cucumber, cut into ribbons 1/2 cup chickpeas, cooked 1 cup sliced cabbage 1/3 cup hummus Mint leaves as needed for topping Hemp seeds as needed for topping 1 bunch of Swiss rainbow chard

Directions: Spread hummus on one side of chard, place some of millet, vegetables, and chickpeas on it, sprinkle with some mint leaves and hemp seeds and wrap it like a burrito. Serve straight away.

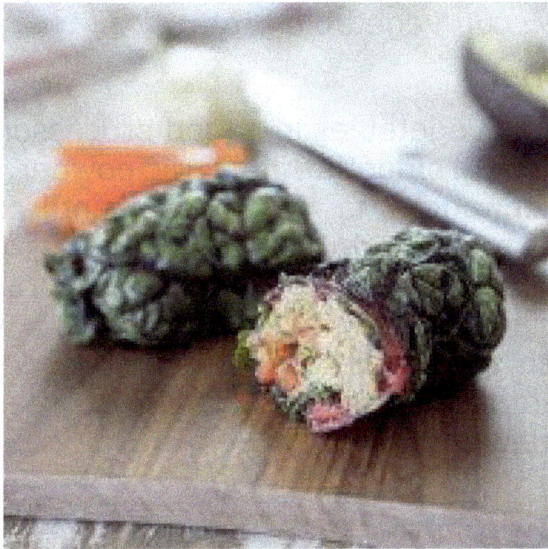

Rice Stuffed Jalapeños

Preparation time: 5 minutes Cooking time: 15 minutes
Servings: 6

Ingredients:

3 medium-sized potatoes, peeled, cubed, boiled 2 large carrots, peeled, chopped, boiled 3 tablespoons water 1/4 teaspoon onion powder 1 teaspoons salt 1/2 cup nutritional yeast 1/4 teaspoon garlic powder 1 lime, juiced 3 tablespoons water Cooked rice as needed 3 jalapeños pepper, halved 1 red bell pepper, sliced, for garnish ½ cup vegetable broth

Directions:

Place boiled vegetables in a food processor, pour in broth and pulse until smooth. Add garlic powder, onion powder, salt, water, and lime juice, pulse until combined, then add yeast and blend until smooth. Tip the mixture in a bowl, add rice, and stir until incorporated. Cut each jalapeno into half lengthwise, brush them with oil, season them with some salt, stuff them with rice mixture and bake them for 20 minutes at 400 degrees F until done. Serve straight away.

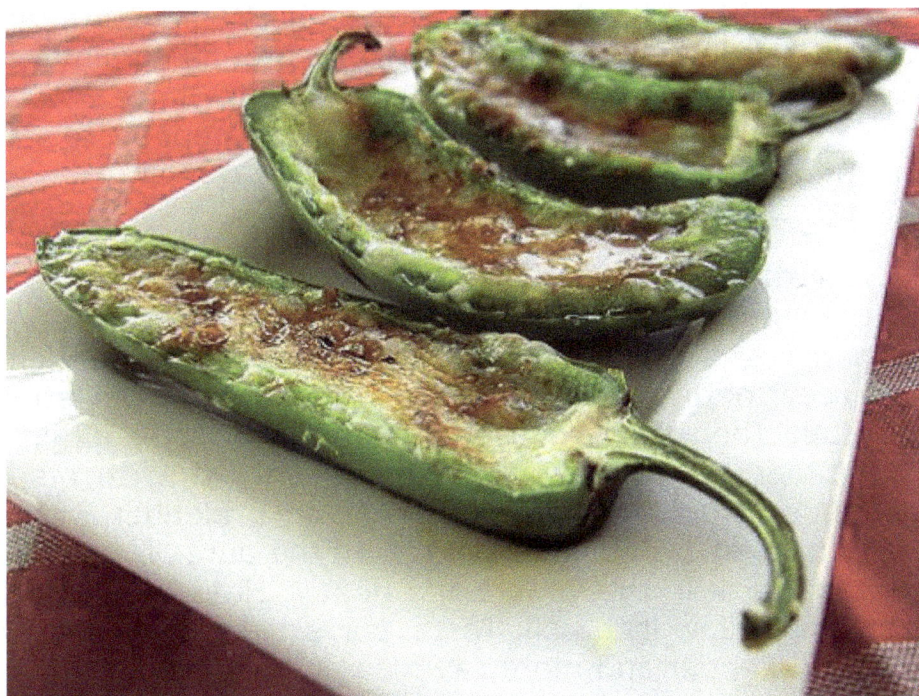

Yogurt Carrot Soup

Preparation time: 5 minutes Cooking time: 50 minutes
Servings: 3

Ingredients:

1 lb. carrots, sliced 2 cups yogurt ½ tsp. ginger ¼ tsp. cayenne pepper 1 onion, peeled and chopped 2 cloves garlic, minced ½ tsp. mustard seeds ½ tsp. turmeric ½ tsp. salt, and more to taste ½ tsp. ground cumin ¼ tsp. cinnamon 4 Tbsp olive oil 1 Tbs. lemon juice 3½ cups water 1 Tbs. honey garnish black pepper to taste chopped fresh cilantro

Directions:

Melt the butter in a skillet and sauté the onions and garlic until they are golden. Add the spices and cook for several minutes, stirring constantly. Add the carrots and lemon juice. Continue cooking for several more minutes, stirring often, then add 2 cups of the water, cover tightly, and simmer for at least ½ hour, or until the carrots are tender. Purée the spiced carrots in a blender with the remaining 1½ cups water. Return the purée to the skillet and whisk in the yogurt and honey. Heat the soup, but do not allow it to boil. Taste, correct the seasoning with black pepper and more cayenne and salt as desired, and serve hot, with chopped cilantro sprinkled on top.

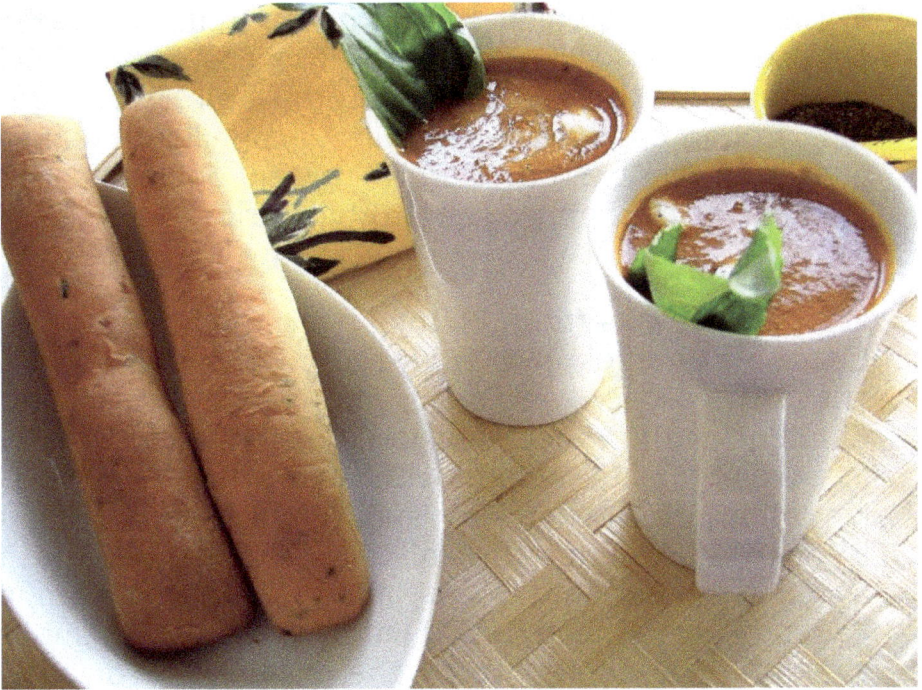

Cold Avocado Soup

Preparation time: 5 minutes Cooking time: 40 minutes
Servings: 3

Ingredients:

2 medium-sized ripe avocados 4 medium-sized tomatoes
½ medium-sized onion 1 clove garlic 1 cucumber 4 Tbs.
chopped green chilis ¾ tsp. salt 3½ Tbs. lemon juice 1
Tbs. red wine vinegar 1 Tbs. vegetable oil 1 tsp. sugar ⅛
tsp. ground cumin 1 cup yogurt ½ cup light cream 1½
cups Vegetable Broth Garnish green onions, chopped
fresh cilantro, chopped fried tortilla strips

Directions:

Peel remove pits from, and coarsely chop the avocados.
Cut the tomatoes in thin wedges. Chop the onion and
mince the garlic. Peel, seed, and cut up the cucumber.
Combine all the vegetables and the chilis and purée them
in a blender until no large chunks are left. Add the salt,
lemon juice, vinegar, oil, sugar, and cumin. Run the
blender again until the mixture is smooth. Pour the
avocado mixture into a bowl, add the yogurt, cream, and
vegetable broth, and beat it lightly with a whisk until it is
smooth once more. Taste the soup and correct the
seasoning if necessary. Chill the soup thoroughly. Chop
up a few green onions and about¼ cup of fresh cilantro
and put them aside in small bowls. Cut several corn
tortillas into short strips and fry them in oil until they are
crisp. Drain them on a paper towel, salt them lightly, and
put them in a napkin-lined bowl or basket. Serve the
soup ice-cold, in chilled bowls if possible, and pass the
onions, cilantro, and tortilla strips separately.

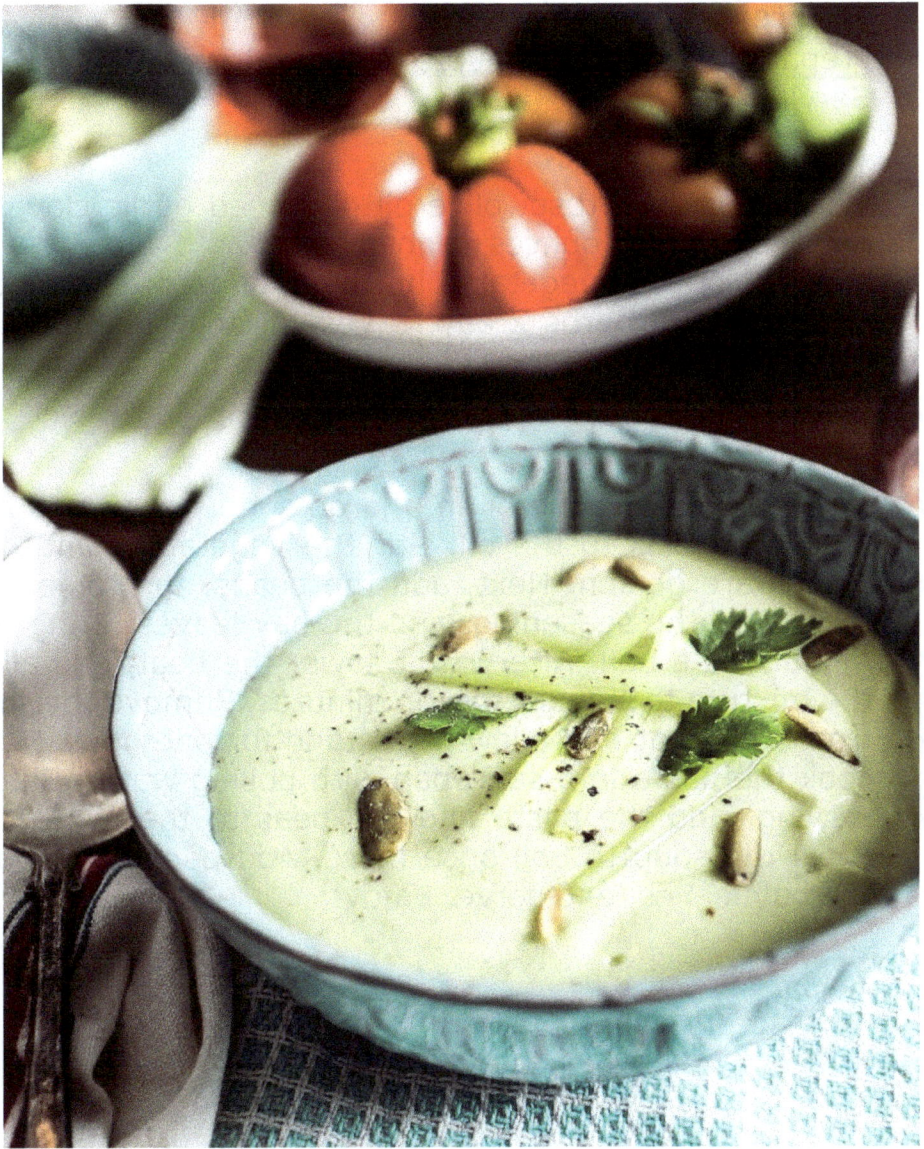

Mediterranean Pasta Soup

Preparation time: 5 minutes Cooking time: 20 minutes 8 Servings.

Ingredients:

1 diced onion 1 tbsp. olive oil 4 minced garlic cloves 1 diced carrot 32 ounces cannellini beans 1 diced celery stalk 32 ounces vegetable broth 16 ounces tomatoes 1 ½ tsp. Italian herbs 2 bay leaves 1 ½ cup peas 2 cups elbow macaroni pasta 1/3 cup minced parsley salt and pepper to taste

Directions:

Begin by heating the oil in a large soup pot and adding the vegetables to the oil. Stir the vegetables until the onions are golden. Next, add the beans, the tomatoes, the broth, the seasoning, and the bay leaves. Bring this mixture to a boil. Afterwards, lower the heat, and allow the mixture to simmer for ten minutes. Remove the soup from the heat and allow it to stand for one hour. Next, cook the pasta in a saucepan with boiling water. Before serving, add the pasta and the peas to the soup, and allow the soup to boil once more. Add parsley, remove the bay leaves, and serve. Enjoy!

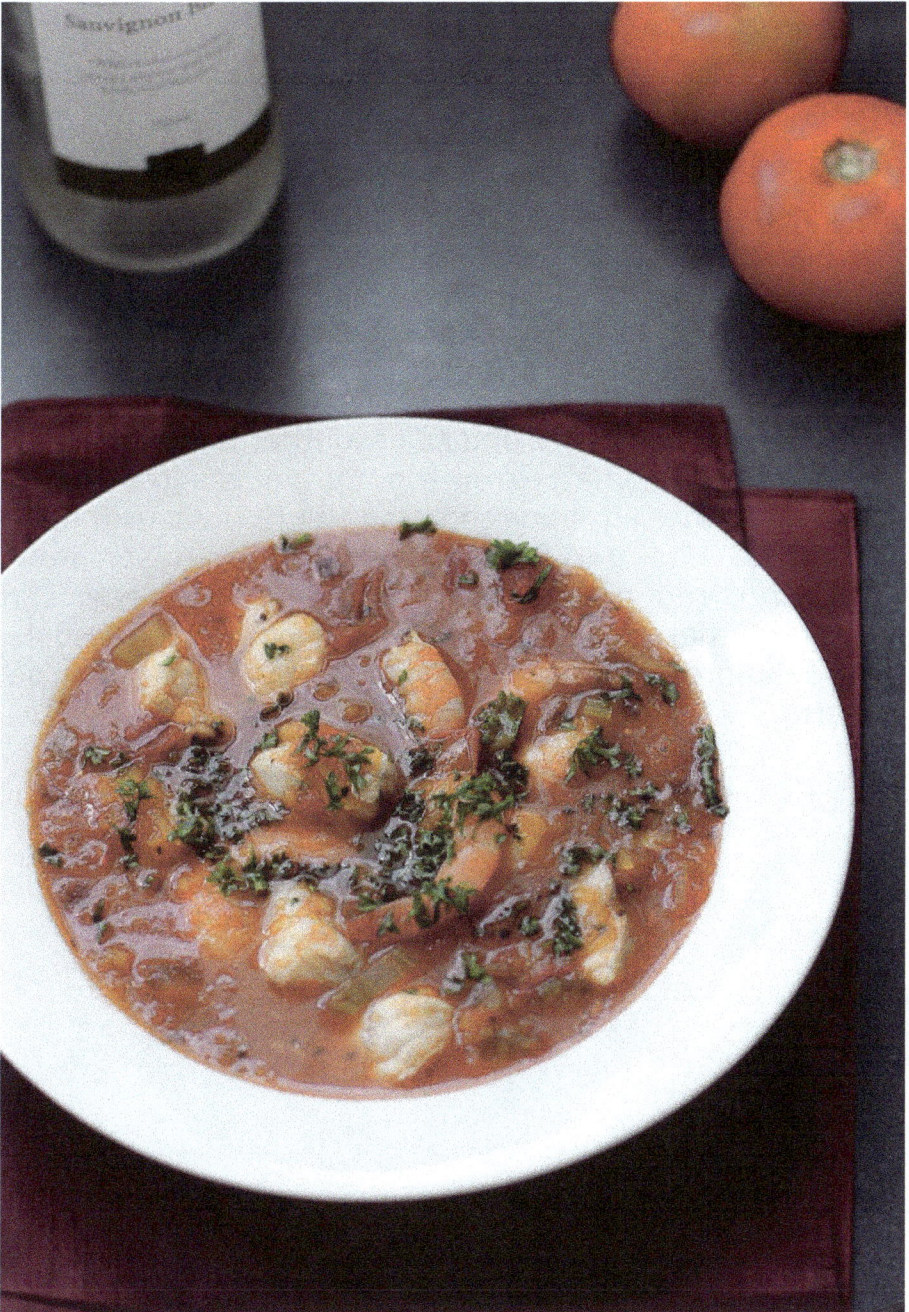

Tomato & Basil Pasta

Preparation time: 5 minutes Cooking time: 20 minutes
Servings: 3

Ingredients:

2 Pinches Red Pepper Flakes 2 Tomatoes, Diced Sea Salt
& Black Pepper to Taste 12 Sweet Basil Leaves, Fresh ½
Teaspoon Garlic Powder ½ Teaspoon Oregano 1 ¾ Cups
Vegetable Stock 2 Cups Campanella Pasta

Directions:

Stir your stock, pasta and salt together in the instant pot,
placing your tomatoes on top. Do not stir the tomatoes
in. Seal the lid and cook on high pressure for two
minutes. Use a quick release, and then stir in your
oregano, red pepper flakes, and garlic powder. Press
sauté if there is still liquid in the bottom and cook for
three more minutes. Stir in the basil and then serve
warm.

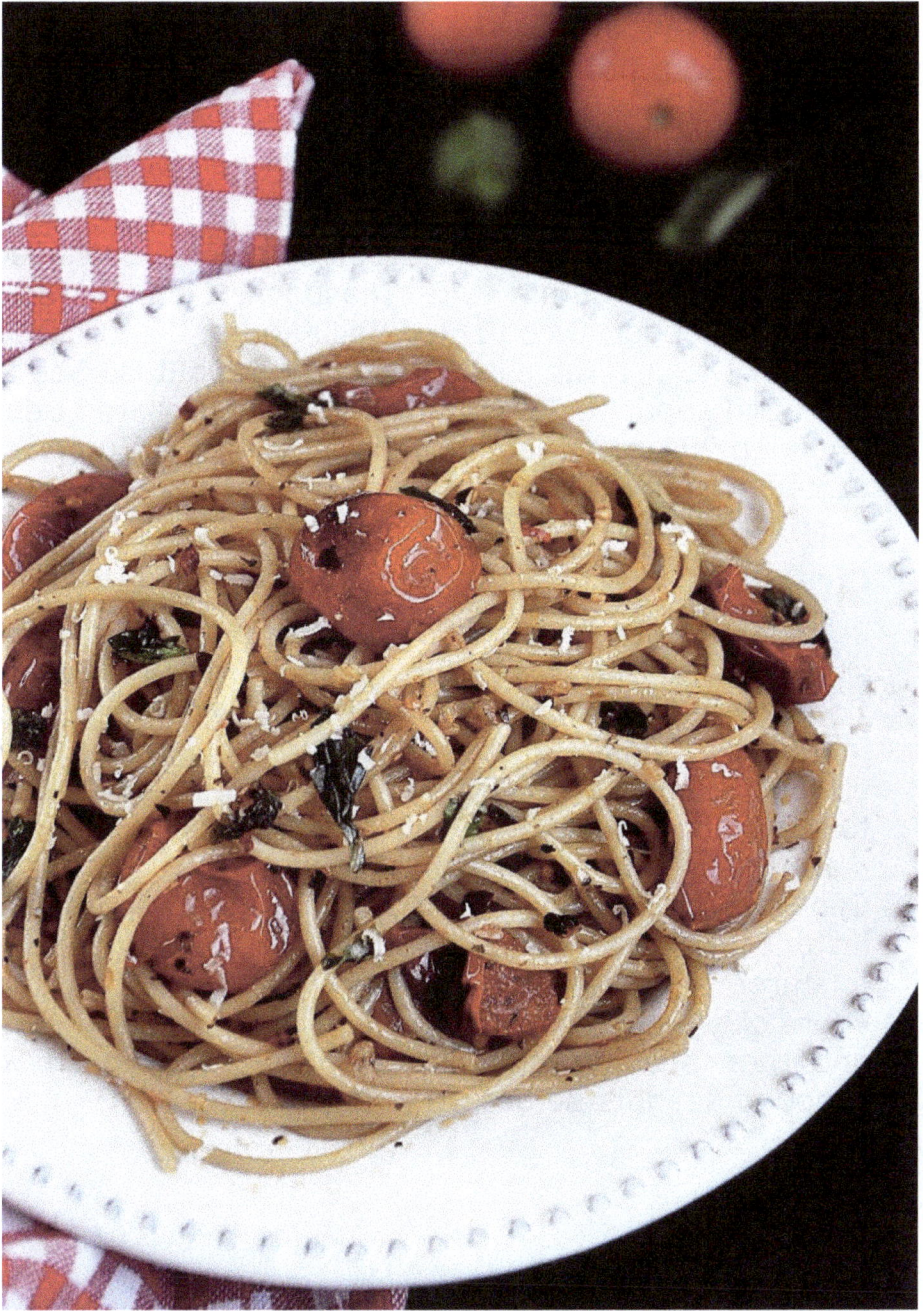

Peanut Stew

Preparation time: 5 minutes Cooking time: 20 minutes
Servings: 4

Ingredients:

3 Cloves Garlic, Minced 3 Tomatoes, Diced 1 Sweet
Potato, Diced 2 Tablespoons Ginger, Peeled & Minced 1
½ Teaspoons Cumin 1/2 Teaspoon Chili Powder 1
Jalapeno Pepper, Diced 1 Red Bell Pepper, Diced 1 Onion,
Small & Diced 1 Tablespoon Roasted Walnut Oil Sea Salt
& Black Pepper to Taste 1 Small Bunch Collard Greens,
Chopped 2 Cups Vegetable Stock, Divided ½ Cup Peanut
Butter, Creamy & Unsweetened ½ Cup Roasted Peanuts,
Chopped

Directions:

Press sauté, and then add in your oil. Once your oil
shimmers add in your onion, jalapeno and bell pepper.
Cook for three minutes, and then add I your garlic. Cook
for another half a minute. Stir in the ginger, cumin,
tomatoes, chili powder, sweet potatoes and salt. Allow it
to rest for a few minutes. Get out a large measuring cup
and whisk your peanut butter with a cup of stock.
Continue to whisk until smooth, and then add it to your
instant pot. Lock the lid, and then cook on high pressure
for three minutes. Use a quick release, and then stir in
your collard greens. Allow them to wilt for two minutes,
and then season with salt and pepper. Garnish with
chopped peanuts before serving.

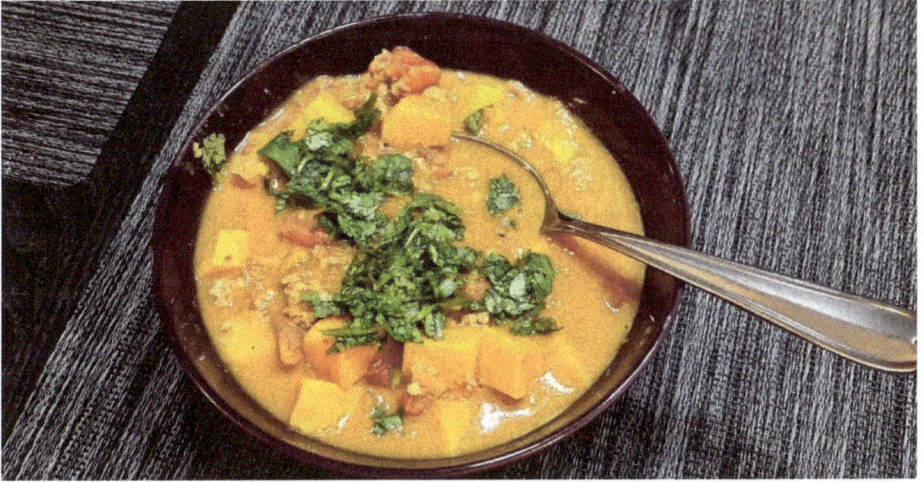

Roasted Leeks and Asparagus

Preparation time: 15 mins Cooking time: 20 minutes
Servings: 12

Ingredients:

3 pounds fresh asparagus, trimmed 2 medium leeks (white portion only), halved lengthwise 1-1/2 teaspoons dill weed 1/2 teaspoon crushed red pepper flakes What you'll need from the store cupboard: 1/4 teaspoon pepper 1/2 teaspoon salt 4 ½ tablespoons olive oil 3 tablespoons melted butter

Directions

Place asparagus and leeks on an ungreased 15x10x1-inch baking pan. Combine the remaining ingredients; pour over vegetables. Bake at 4000F for 20-25 minutes or until tender, stirring occasionally.

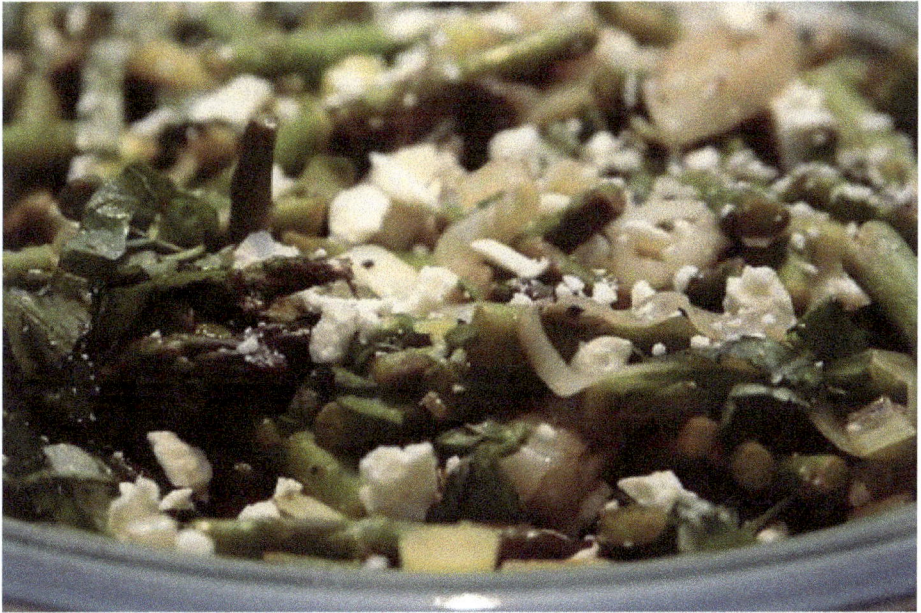

Guacamole

Preparation time: 10 minutes Cooking time: 0 minutes
Servings: 2

Ingredients:

2 medium ripe avocados 1 tablespoon lemon juice 1/4
cup chopped tomatoes 4 tablespoons olive oil What you'll
need from the store cupboard: 1/4 teaspoon salt Pepper
to taste

Directions:

Peel and chop avocados; place in a small bowl. Sprinkle
with lemon juice. Add salsa and salt. Season with pepper
to taste and mash coarsely with a fork. Refrigerate until
serving.

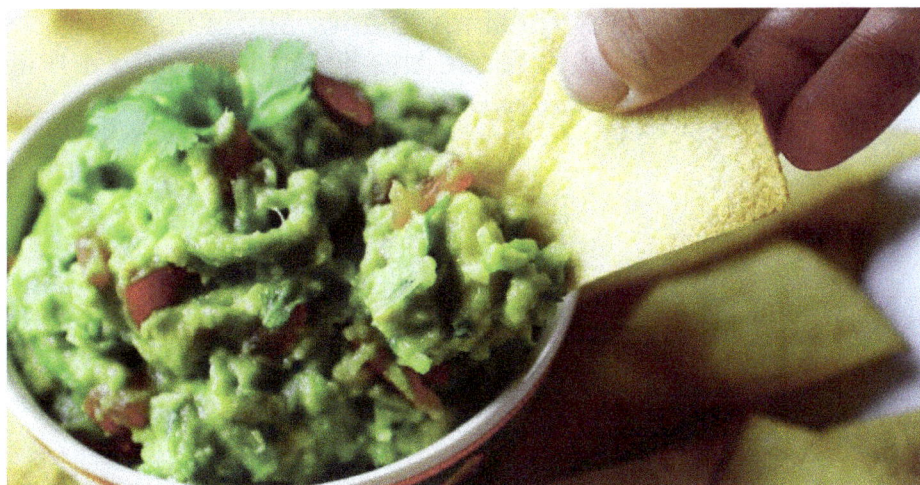

Butternut Squash and Cauliflower Stew

Prep time: 5 minutes Cooking time:10 minutes Servings: 4

Ingredients:

3 cloves of garlic, minced 1 cup cauliflower florets 1 ½ cups butternut squash, cubed 2 ½ cups heavy cream What you'll need from the store cupboard: Pepper and salt to taste 3 tbsp coconut oil

Directions

Heat the oil in a pan and saute the garlic until fragrant. Stir in the rest of the ingredients and season with salt and pepper to taste. Close the lid and bring to a boil for 10 minutes. Serve and enjoy.

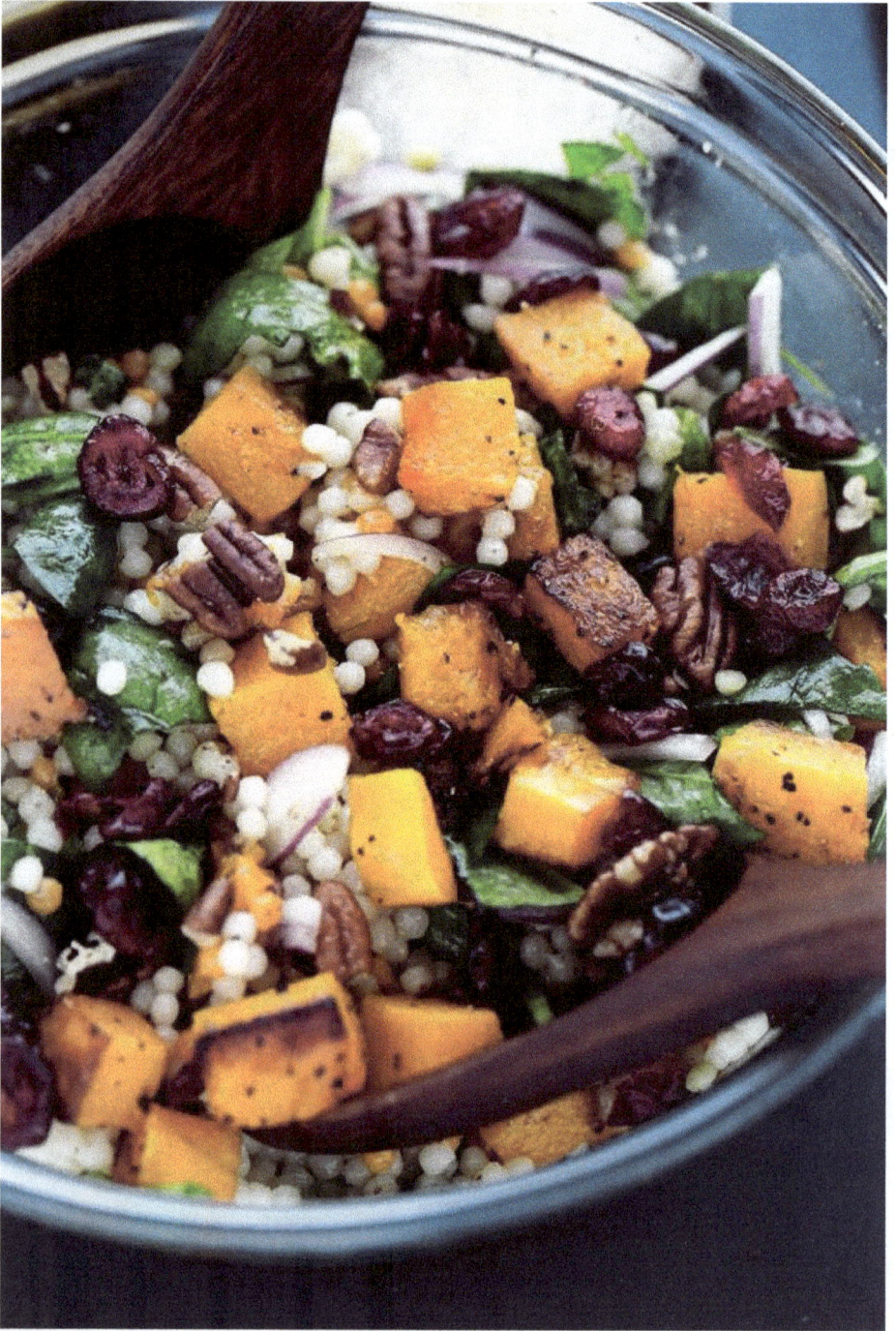

Greek Styled Veggie-Rice

Preparation time: 15 minutes Cooking time: 20 minutes
Servings: 3

Ingredients:

3 tbsp chopped fresh mint 1 small tomato, chopped 1
head cauliflower, cut into large florets ¼ cup fresh lemon
juice ½ yellow onion, minced What you'll need from the
store cupboard: pepper and salt to taste ¼ cup extra
virgin olive oil

Directions

In a bowl, mix lemon juice and onion and leave for 30
minutes. Then drain onion and reserve the juice and
onion bits. In a blender, shred cauliflower until the size
of a grain of rice. On medium fire, place a medium
nonstick skillet and for 8-10 minutes cook cauliflower
while covered. Add grape tomatoes and cook for 3
minutes while stirring occasionally. Add mint and onion
bits. Cook for another three minutes. Meanwhile, in a
small bowl whisk pepper, salt, 3 tbsp reserved lemon
juice, and olive oil until well blended. Remove cooked
cauliflower, transfer to a serving bowl, pour lemon juice
mixture, and toss to mix. Before serving, if needed
season with pepper and salt to taste.

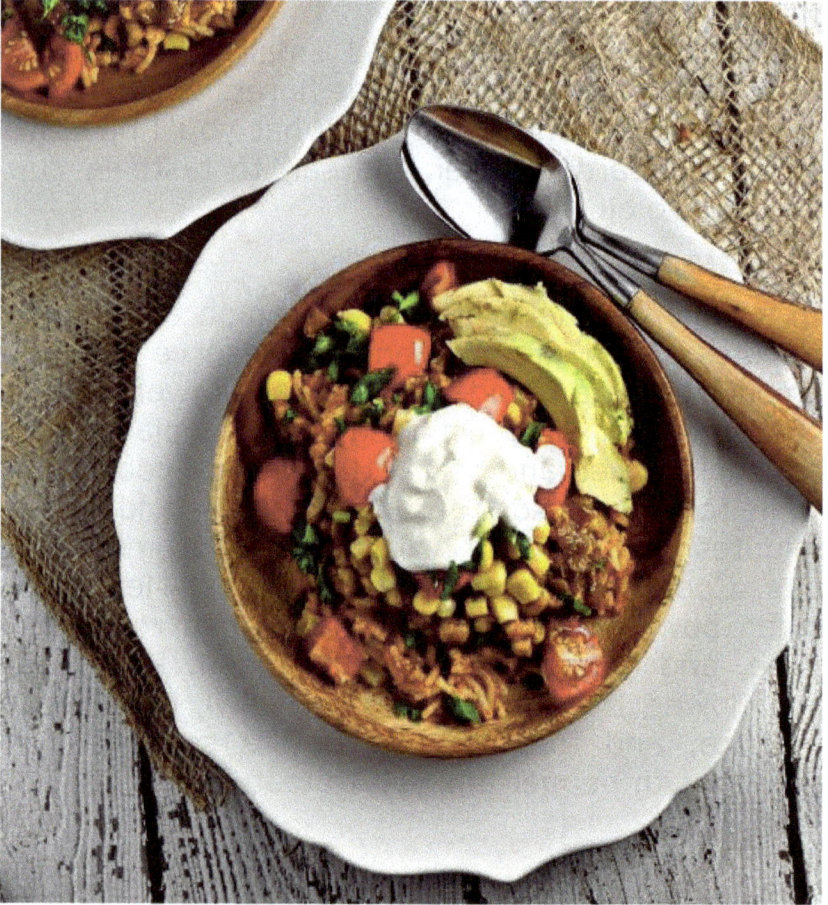

Garlic 'n Sour Cream Zucchini Bake

Preparation time: minutesCooking time: 20 minutes Servings: 3

Ingredients:

1 ½ cups zucchini slices 5 tablespoons olive oil 1 tablespoon minced garlic 1/4 cup grated Parmesan cheese 1 (8 ounces) package cream cheese, softened What you'll need from the store cupboard: Salt and pepper to taste

Directions

Lightly grease a baking sheet with cooking spray. Place zucchini in a bowl and put in olive oil and garlic. Place zucchini slices in a single layer in dish. Bake for 35 minutes at 390oF until crispy. In a bowl, whisk well, remaining ingredients. Serve with zucchini.

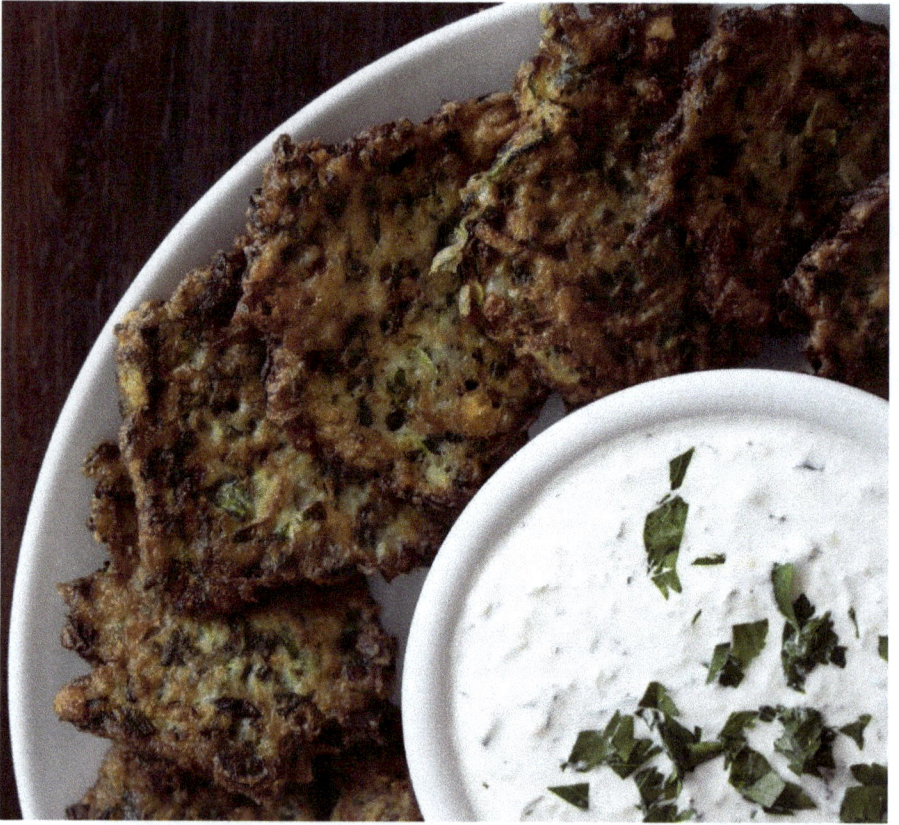

Leek & Potato Soup

Preparation time: 5 minutes Cooking time: 30 minutes Servings: 4

Ingredients:

4 Cups Vegetable Stock 1 lb. Gold Potatoes, Cubed 1 Bay Leaf ½ Teaspoon Sea Salt, Fine 2/3 Cup Soy Milk 2 Cloves Garlic, Minced 2 Leeks, Chopped 3 Tablespoons Vegan Butter Black Pepper to Taste 1/3 Cup Olive Oil

Directions:

Press sauté, and then select low. Once it's hot, add in your butter. Once your butter has melted, add in your leaks and cook until soft. Stir occasionally. This should take three minutes, and then add in your garlic. Cook for half a minute. Pour in the bay leaf, potatoes, stock and salt. Stir well, and then cook on high pressure for five minutes. Use a natural pressure release for fifteen minutes, and then use a quick release for any remaining pressure. Combine your olive oil and soy milk together in a blender, and blend until smooth. This will make a substitute for heavy cream. Discard the bay leaf and add in your substitute cream. Use an immersion blender to blend until smooth.

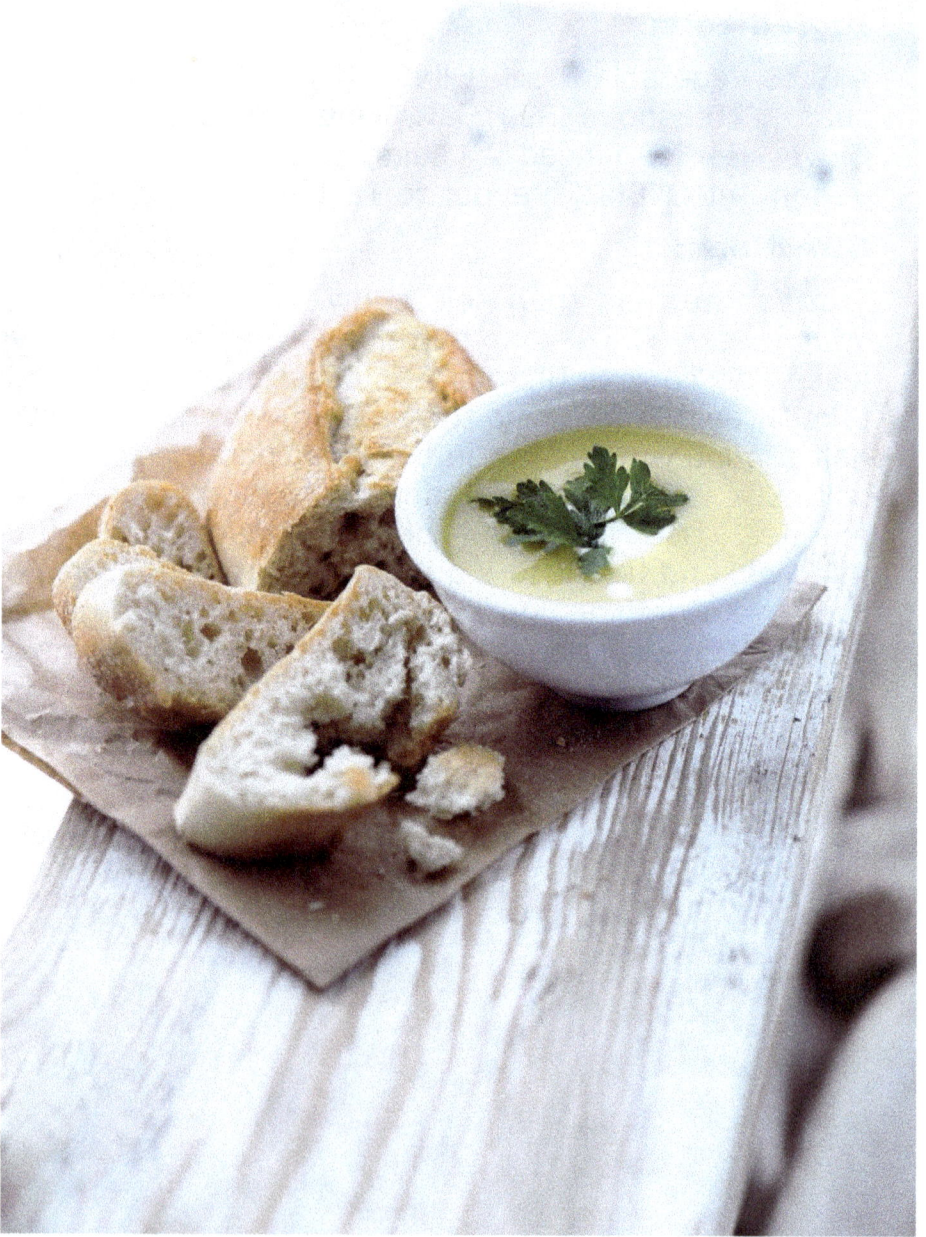

Tomato & Tofu Bake

Preparation time: 5 minutes Cooking time: 25 minutes
Servings: 4

Ingredients:

2 Tablespoons Banana Pepper Rings, Canned ½ Cup
Vegetable Broth 14.5 Ounces Tomatoes, Canned & Diced
with Juices 1 Block Tofu, Crumbled 1 Tablespoons Italian
Seasoning

Directions:

Combine all of your ingredients and seal the lid. Cook for
four minutes on high pressure, and then use a quick
release. Serve warm.

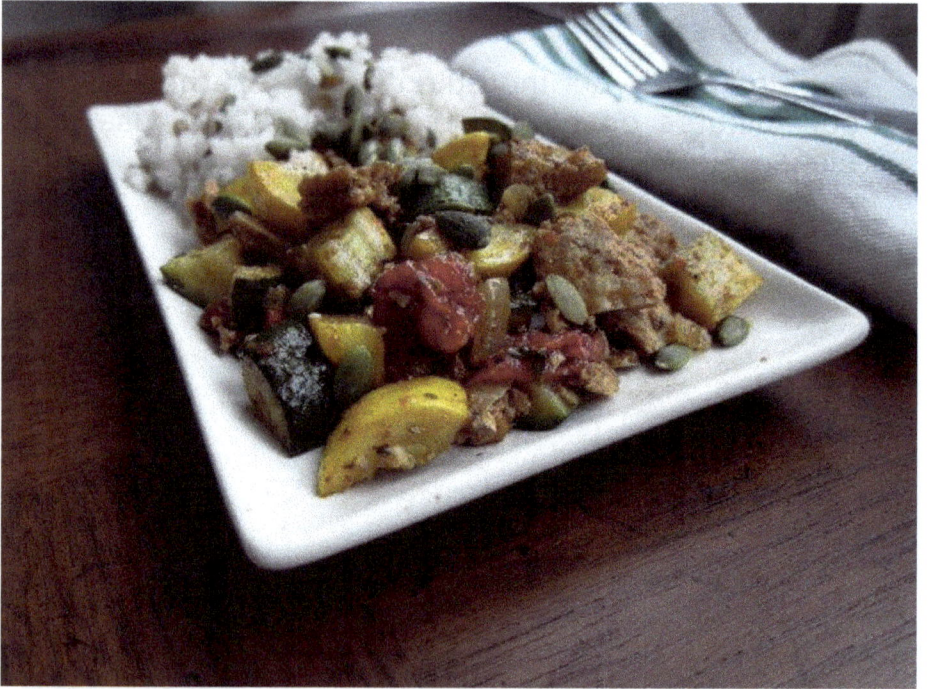

Cream of Mushroom Soup

Preparation time: 5 minutes Cooking time: 20 minutes Servings: 4

Ingredients:

1 ¾ Cup Vegetable Stock ½ Cup Silken Tofu 1 Teaspoon Sea Salt, Fine 2 Cloves Garlic, Minced 2 Teaspoons Thyme 1 ½ lbs. White Button Mushrooms, Sliced 1 Sweet Onion, Small & Chopped 2 Tablespoons Vegan Butter Thyme, Fresh & Chopped for Garnish

Directions: Press sauté and place it on low. Once it's hot, add in your butter. Once your butter has melted add in your onion, and cook for two minutes. Throw in the thyme, salt, mushrooms and garlic. Cook for two more minutes, and then stir in your stock. Lock the lid, and then cook on high pressure for six minutes. Put your tofu in a blender, and blend until smooth. Set the blended tofu aside, and then then allow for a natural pressure release for ten minutes. Use a quick release for any remaining pressure. Use an immersion blender, and blend until creamy. Stir in the tofu, and garnish before serving.

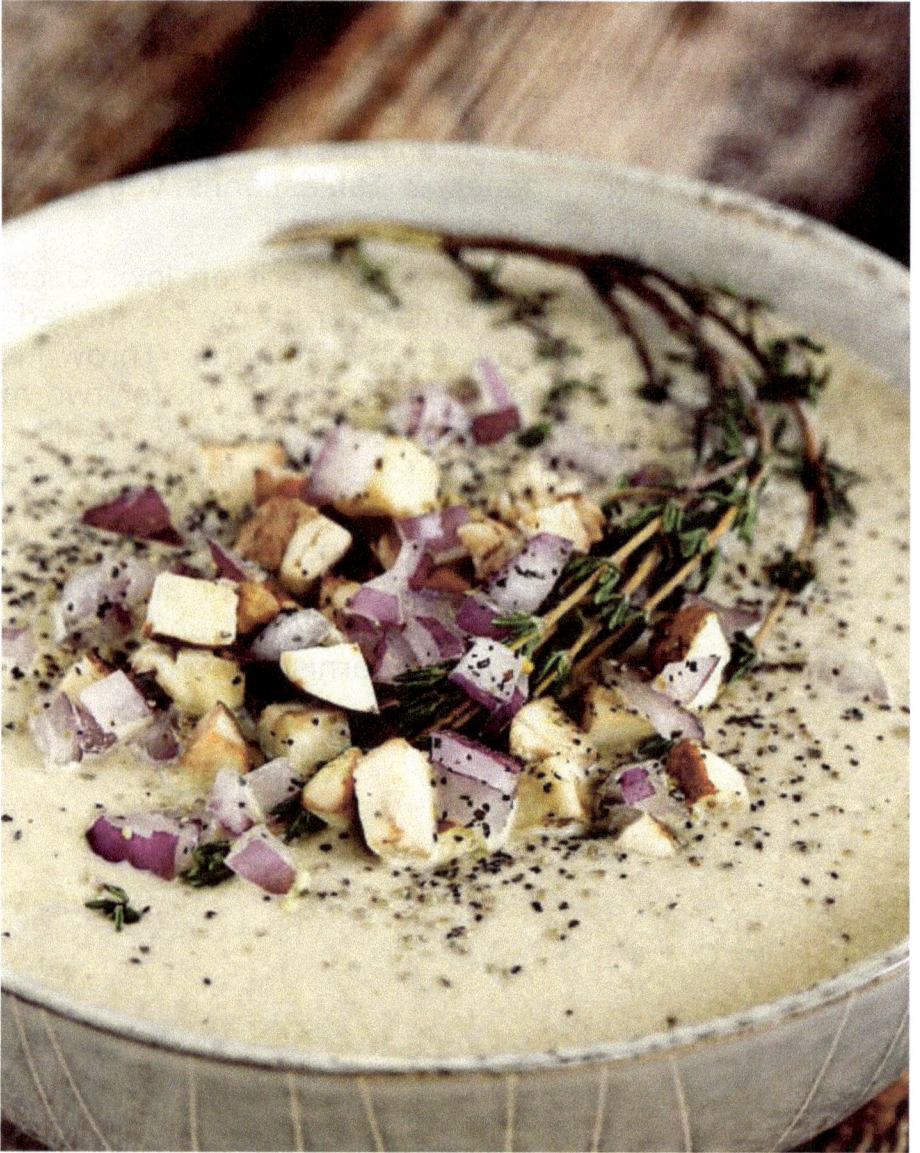

Moroccan Split Pea Soup

Preparation time: 5 minutes Cooking time: 20 minutes
Servings: 8

Ingredients:

1 Cup Split Peas, Rinsed 3 Stalks Celery 2 Carrots,
Chopped 4 Spring Onions, Chopped 1 Bell Pepper,
Chopped 6 Cups Vegetable Stock 14 Ounces Tomatoes,
Chopped Fine 1 Teaspoon Cinnamon 1 Teaspoon Ground
Coriander 1 Teaspoon Smoked Paprika 1 Teaspoon
Garlic, Minced 1 Teaspoon Cumin Sea Salt & Black Pepper
to Taste

Directions:

Throw all of your ingredients into the instant pot and stir.
Cook on high pressure for twelve minutes. If you want
your peas to be softer, cook for fifteen minutes more.
Use a natural pressure release for five minutes, and then
use a quick release for any remaining pressure. Stir well,
and allow it to settle to thicken before serving warm.

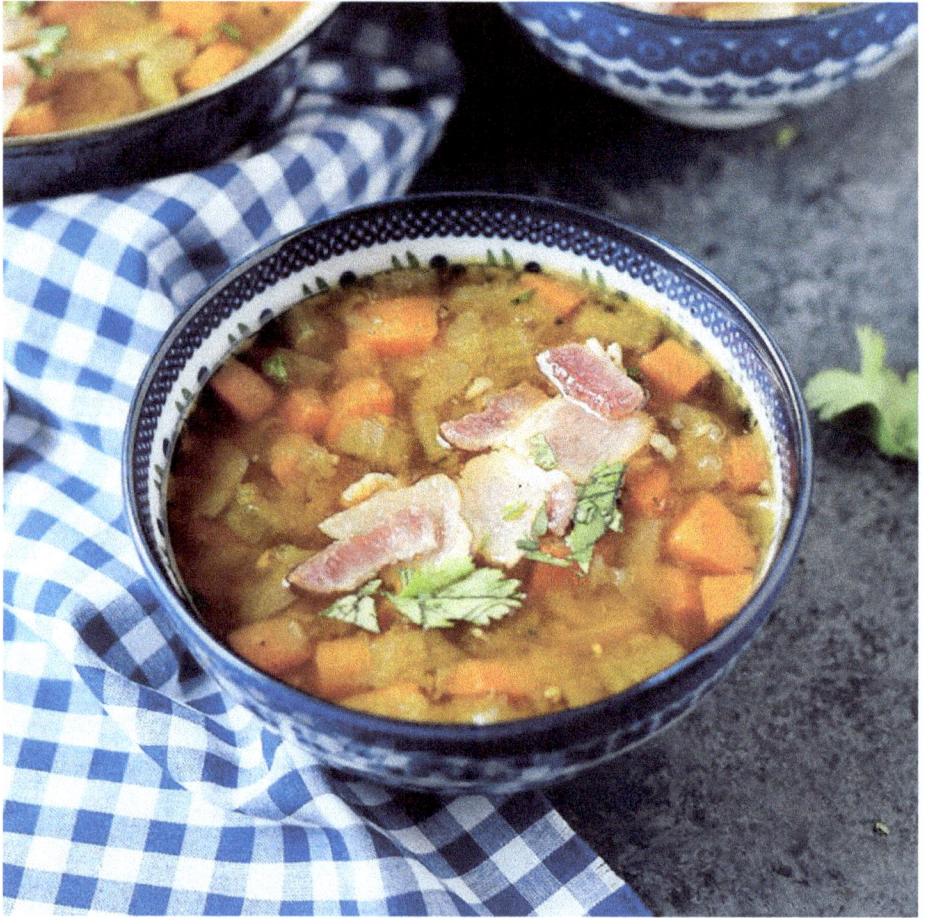

Curried Squash Soup

Preparation time: 5 minutes Cooking time: 60 minutes
Servings: 4

Ingredients:

1 Tablespoons Olive Oil 1 Onion, Chopped 2 Cloves
Garlic, Chopped 1 Tablespoon Curry Powder 3 lbs.
Butternut Squash, Peeled & Cubed Sea Salt & Black
Pepper to Taste 4 Cups Vegetable Stock 14 Ounces
Coconut Milk, Canned & Lite

Directions:

Press sauté, and then once it's hot add in your oil. When
your oil begins to shimmer, add in the onion and cook for
four minutes. Add the curry powder and garlic, and then
cook for another minute while stirring. Add in your stock,
squash and salt. Seal the lid, and cook on high pressure
for thirty minutes. Use a quick release, and then use an
immersion blender to blend until smooth. Stir in the
coconut milk, but save a little for topping when serving.

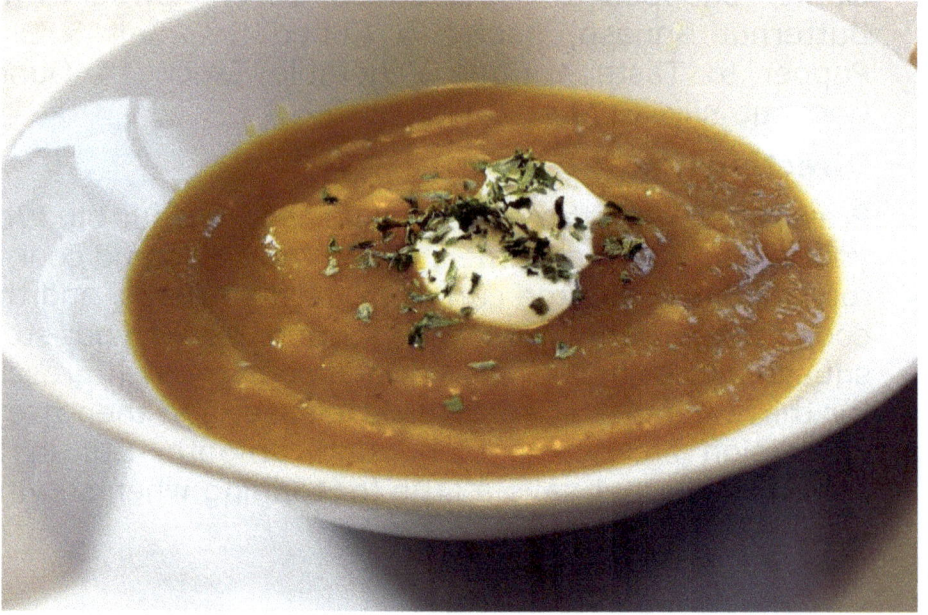

Curried Lentil Soup

Preparation time: 5 minutes Cooking time: 30 minutes
Servings: 5-6

Ingredients:

1 cup dried lentils 1 large onion, finely cut 1 celery rib,
chopped 1 large carrot, chopped 3 garlic cloves, chopped
1 can tomatoes, undrained 3 cups vegetable broth 1 tbsp
curry powder 1/2 tsp ground ginger

Directions:

Combine all ingredients in slow cooker. Cover and cook
on low for 5-6 hours. Blend soup to desired consistency,
adding additional hot water to thin, if desired.

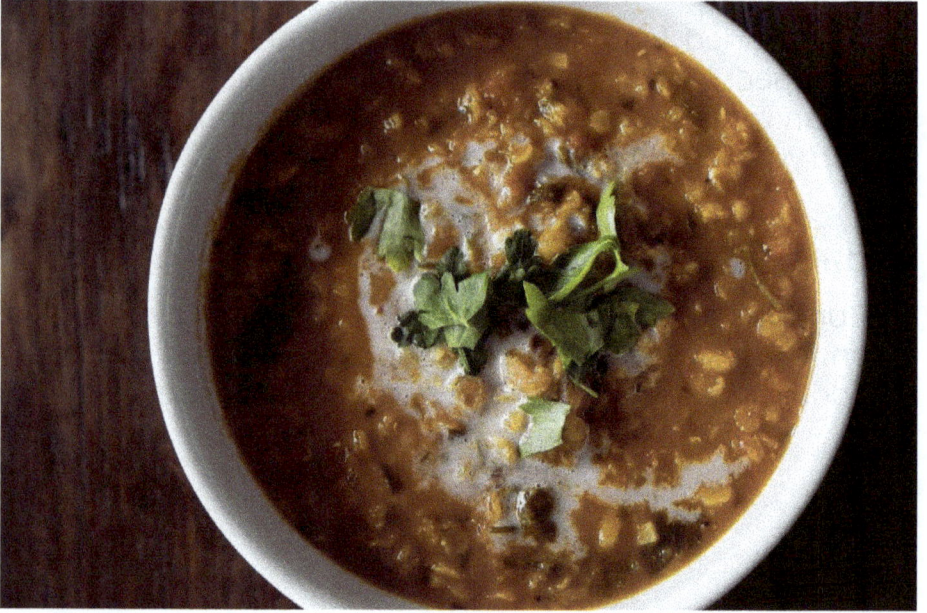

Simple Black Bean Soup

Preparation time: 5 minutes Cooking time: 50 minutes
Servings: 5-6

Ingredients:

1 cup dried black beans 5 cups vegetable broth 1 large
onion, chopped 1 red pepper, chopped 1 tsp sweet
paprika 1 tbsp dried mint 2 bay leaves 1 Serrano chili,
finely chopped 1 tsp salt 4 tbsp fresh lime juice 1/2 cup
chopped fresh cilantro 1 cup vegan cream, to serve

Directions:

Wash the beans and soak them in enough water
overnight. In a slow cooker, combine the beans and all
other ingredients except for the lime juice and cilantro.
Cover and cook on low for 7-8 hours. Add salt, lime juice
and fresh cilantro. Serve with a dollop of vegan cream.

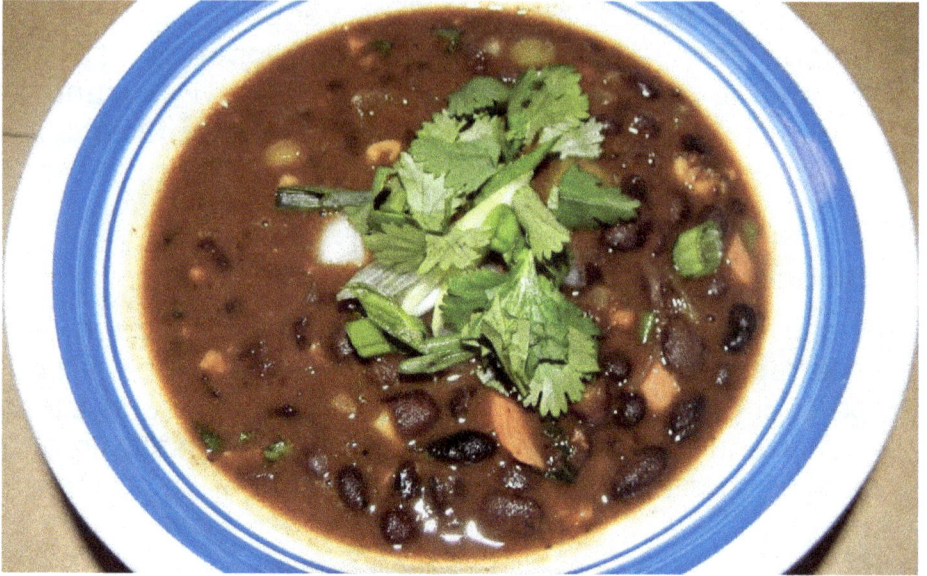

Slow Cooked Split Pea Soup

Preparation time: 5 minutes Cooking time: 50 minutes
Servings: 5-6

Ingredients:

1 lb dried green split peas, rinsed and drained 2 potatoes, peeled and diced 1 small onion, chopped 1 celery rib, chopped 1 carrot, chopped 2 garlic cloves, chopped 1 bay leaf 1 tsp black pepper 1/2 tsp salt 6 cups water

Directions:

Combine all ingredients in slow cooker. Cover and cook on low for 5-6 hours. Discard bay leaf. Blend soup to desired consistency, adding additional hot water to thin, if desired. Serve with garlic or herb bread.

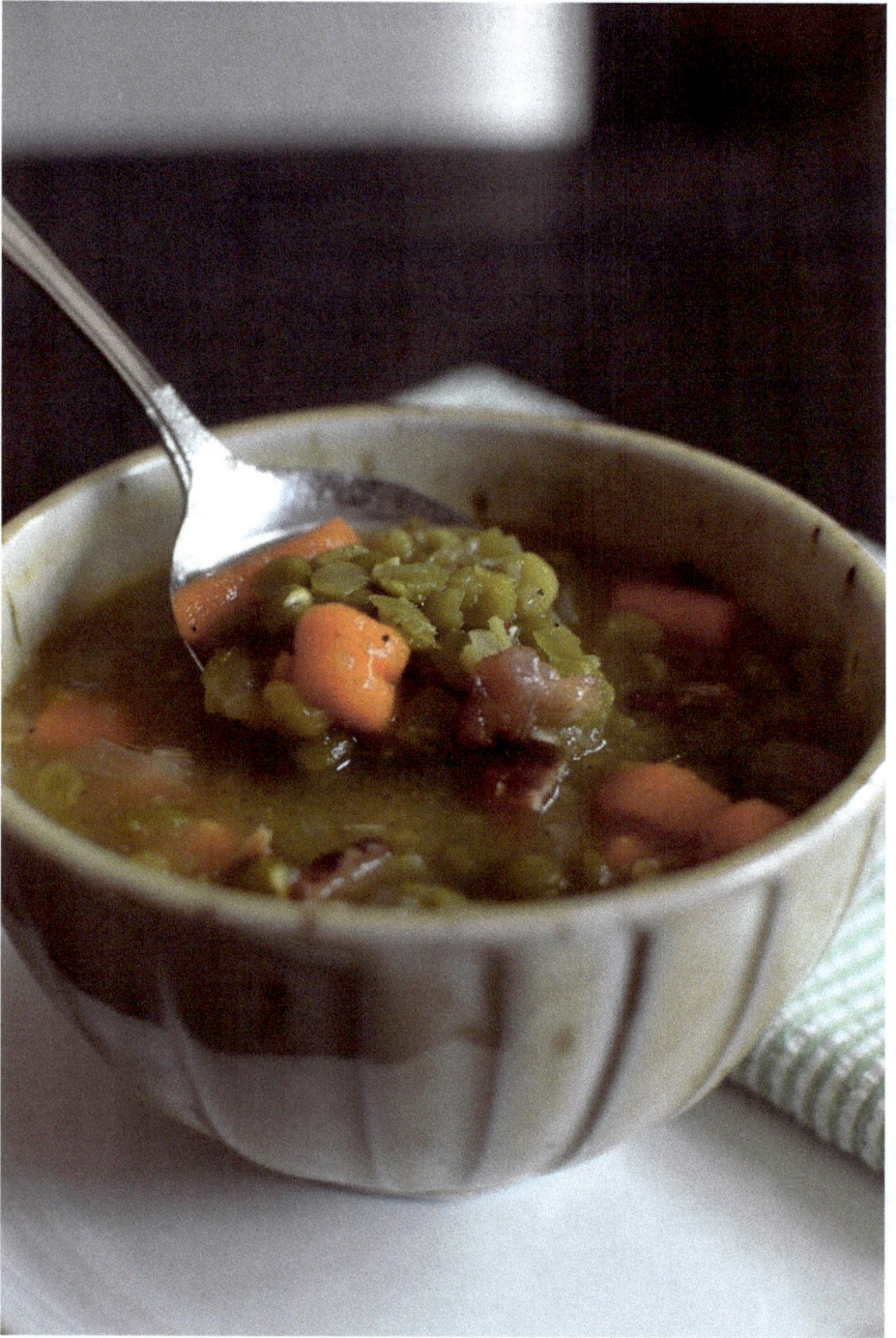

Slow Cooker Tuscan-style Soup

Preparation time: 5 minutes Cooking time: 20 minutes
Servings: 5-6

Ingredients:

1 lb potatoes, peeled and cubed 1 small onion, chopped
1 can mixed beans, drained 1 carrot, chopped 2 garlic
cloves, chopped 4 cups vegetable broth 1 cups chopped
kale 3 tbsp olive oil 1 bay leaf salt and pepper, to taste
Grated vegan cheese, to serve

Directions:

Heat oil in a skillet over medium heat and sauté the
onion, carrot and garlic, stirring, for 2-3 minutes or until
soft. Combine all ingredients except the kale into the slow
cooker. Season with salt and pepper to taste. Cook on
high for 4 hours or low for 6-7 hours. Add in kale about
30 minutes before soup is finished cooking. Serve
sprinkled with vegan cheese.

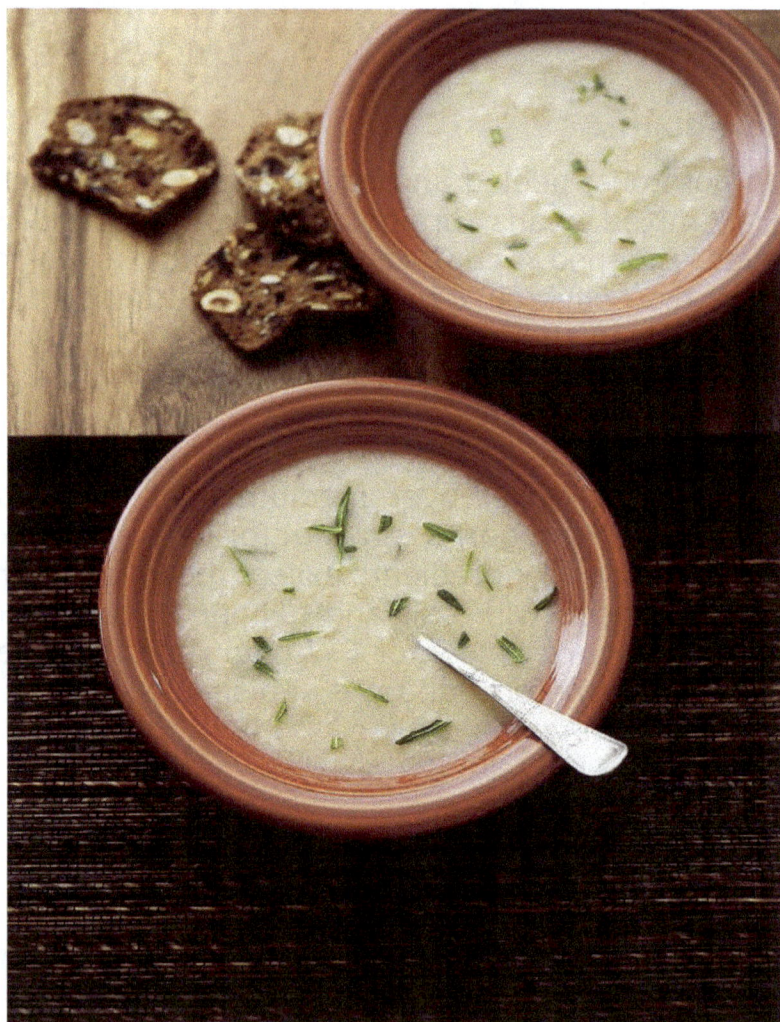

Vitamin C-Stocked Barley Soup

Preparation time: 5 minutes Cooking time: 60 minutes 10 cups.

Ingredients:

2 diced onions 1 tbsp. olive oil 4 minced garlic cloves 4 diced green onions 2 diced zucchinis 1 diced yellow pepper 3 diced carrots 5 cups vegetable broth 20 ounces diced tomatoes ½ cup buckwheat groats 1/3 cup pearled barley 2 tbsp. lemon juice 3 tbsp. parsley salt and pepper to taste

Directions:

Begin by heating the onion, the garlic, and the olive oil in the bottom of a large soup pot. Heat them for eight minutes. Next, add the spices and cook for an additional two minutes. Add the rest of the vegetables, and cook them for five more minutes. Next, add the broth, the diced tomatoes, the buckwheat, and the barley. Allow the soup to simmer for twenty minutes. Make sure to stir it every few moments. Next, add the lemon juice and the rest of the spices you desire. Cook the mixture for a few more minutes, stirring occasionally. Then, serve warm, and enjoy!

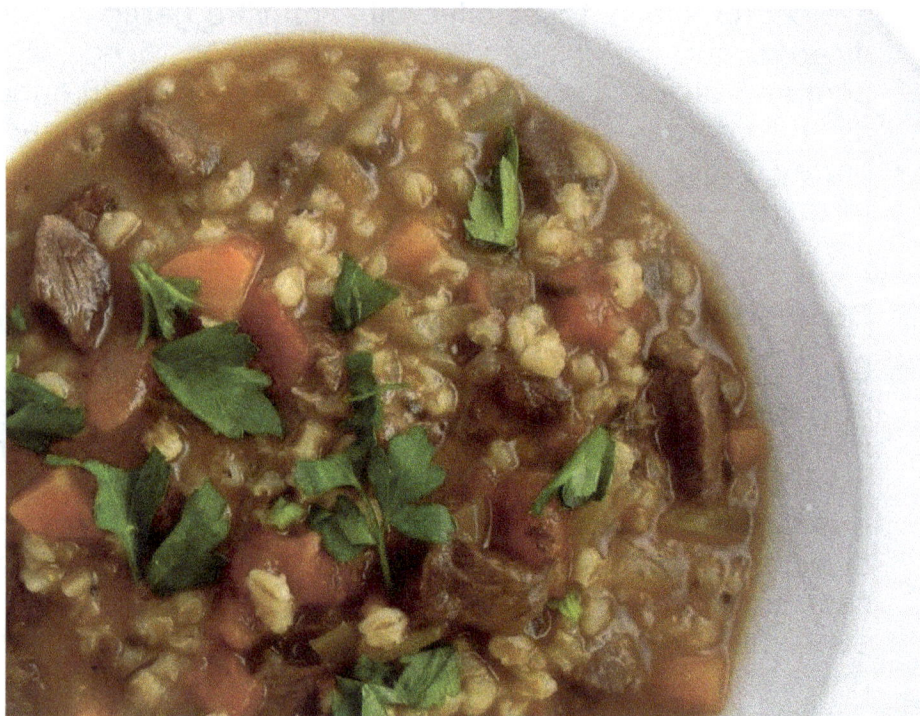

www.ingramcontent.com/pod-product-compliance
Lightning Source LLC
Chambersburg PA
CBHW050754030426
42336CB00012B/1820